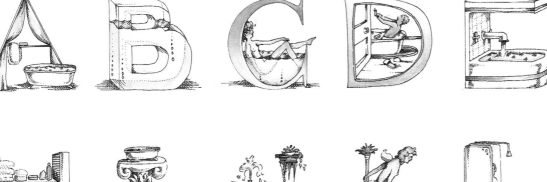

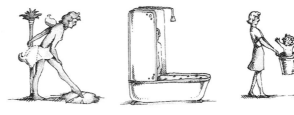
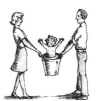
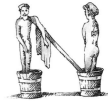

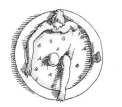
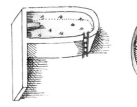
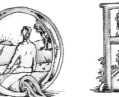
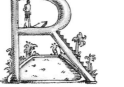
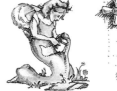
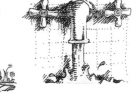
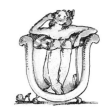

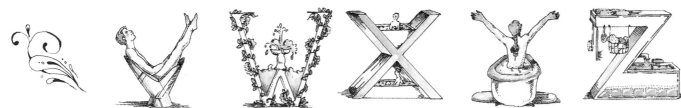

THE BOOK OF THE BATH

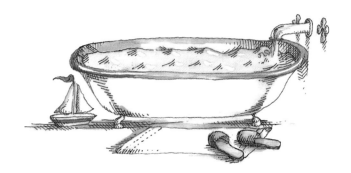

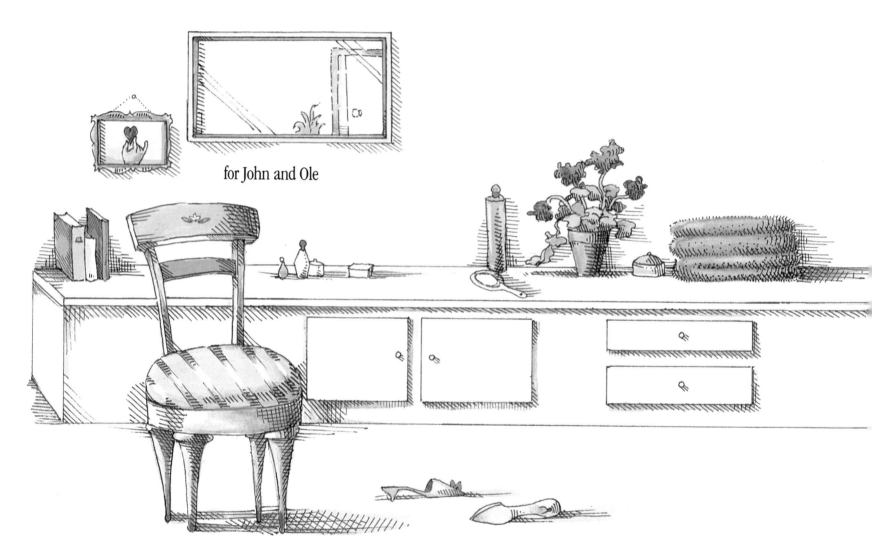

for John and Ole

The Book Of The Bath

Written and Illustrated by
Catherine Kanner

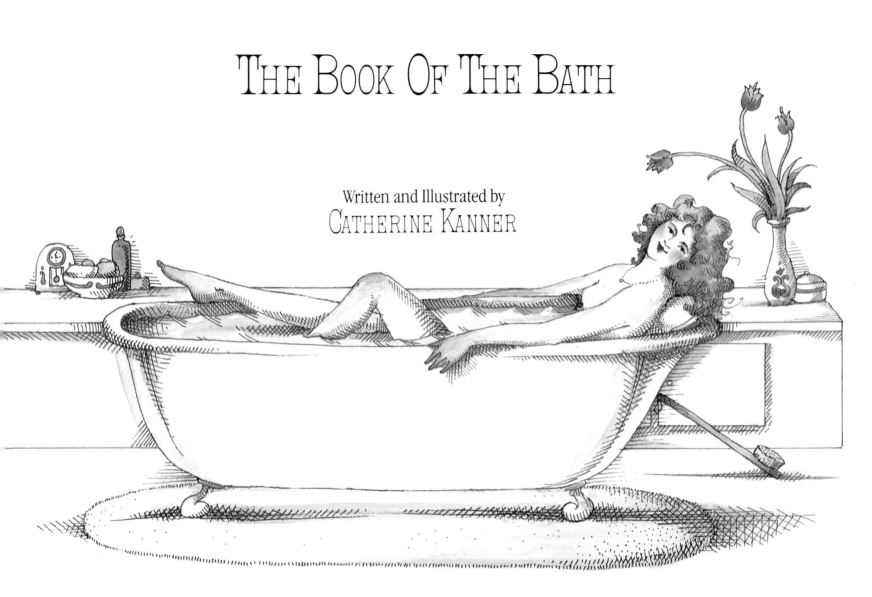

FAWCETT COLUMBINE • NEW YORK

ACKNOWLEDGMENTS

The author wishes to acknowledge Joëlle Delbourgo for her enthusiasm and guidance, and Sarah Mollman for her devotion to every detail in the production of this book. Special thanks to John Locke for his unwaivering support, and Ole Risom for his belief in the project.

Appreciation to Jasper Rose for his ever-present inspiration. Thanks to Rob and Susan. And special thanks to my Parents and Stephen who taught me about beauty.

A Fawcett Columbine Book

Published by Ballantine Books

Library of Congress Catalog Card Number: 85-90573
ISBN 0-449- 90165-3

Manufactured in the United States of America
First Edition: October 1985
10 9 8 7 6 5 4 3 2 1

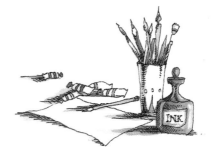

CONTENTS

About the Bath

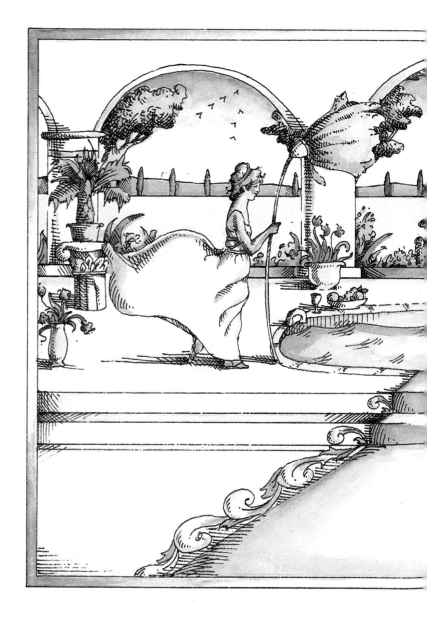

We are born into this world after the longest, most wonderful warm bath of all. No matter who you are or where you live, you have taken a bath. You know the sound of water rushing in the tub, the steam on the mirror, the scent of the soap. You settle into the warmth surrounding you, and the tensions of the day fall away. It is a moment of pure pleasure and well-being. The bath.

I have loved baths for as long as I can remember. When I was a child, the only bathtub in our house was a beautiful porcelain basin with claw feet. It was the exclusive property of my mother, who adored it. Everyone else showered. Only when I had been especially good was I treated to a bath, which was sometimes scented with lavender or had rose petals floating in it. This is where I first learned to appreciate the finer aspects of bathing. Many baths later, I was inspired to write this book. As you read, I hope, you

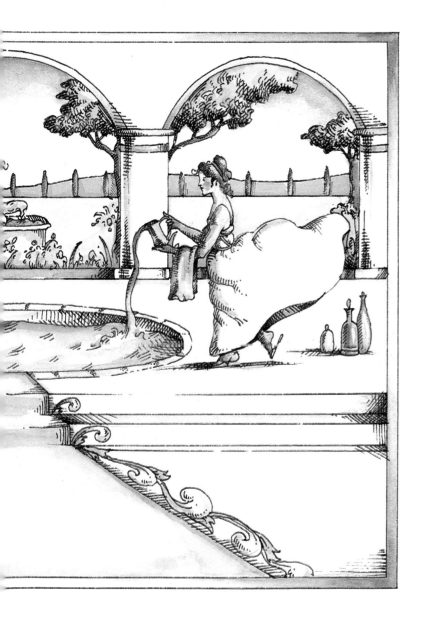

will see that a good bath is about more than just getting clean. It is about privacy, renewal, and the joy of maintaining a healthy body and spirit.

Today you and I have the luxury of hot water from the tap and entire rooms for the indulgence of a bath. But this was not always so. People's bathing habits were determined by a number of limitations and nuisances, not the least of which was an aversion to getting wet. Man's first baths were probably accidental and cold. The habit of cleansing wounds in fresh running streams had to be learned from animals. Primitive families in all cultures bathed together, sharing the same basin or watering place. Since it was difficult to heat quantities of water, people took cold baths. Soap was unpopular. For most people bathing was a disagreeable chore, and it was easier to remain stinking than to take the plunge. There were sublime exceptions, however.

The Greeks and Romans were the first to bathe regularly in cold water. The first bath resorts were built near natural springs. These resorts offered spiritual as well as physical cures. Water was thought to be the essence of life. Homer considered it the principle of all things.

"And the men themselves waded into the sea and washed off the dense sweat from skin and shoulder and thigh. Afterwards...when...the inward heart had been cooled to refreshment they stepped into the bathtubs smooth-polished, and bathed there, and after they had bathed and anointed themselves with olive oil they sat down to dine..."
—ILIAD

Hippocrates was a great believer in cold water cures, and used them in the treatment of the most serious illnesses.

Private baths in early times were more ritual than hygienic. Upon arriving at the home of a wealthy friend, a guest was greeted and escorted to a room where, aided by a handmaiden, his skin would be scraped with an iron utensil (in lieu of soap) and then drenched with an urn of cold water. Ritual bathing such as this occurs throughout history and across cultures.

In the 5th century B.C., the Greeks built small luxurious bath houses for men and women. Soap was first used at this time. It was made of goat's fat and ashes and was quite unpopular. The Greeks preferred sponges, oils, scrapers, and rinses to maintain a healthy glow.

The Romans were famous for taking baths. Some say Rome fell because too many people spent too much time in the public baths! The first Roman bath houses appeared around 312 B.C., when aqueducts made water more accessible. In the warm Roman climate, the baths were a welcome convenience.

The thermae (bath houses) offered a variety of hot water delights. It was the custom to strip, exercise and steam in a hot room, then take a warm bath and finish with a dip in a cold water pool.

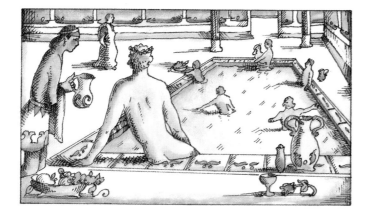

This sounds like the health spas we enjoy today, with the difference that slaves were retained to stoke fires, scrape, anoint, massage, perfume, and generally attend to the whims of the bather. After a bath, Romans could choose from a wide variety of scents and perfumes. A taste for luxury had overtaken the simple pleasures of bathing.

There were 952 baths in 4th century B.C. Rome. The largest of these contained lecture rooms, libraries, and huge pools. Walls were lavishly covered with Egyptian marble, ornamental stone and glass, and exquisite frescoes. Women began bathing with men, and thus began a scandalous era.

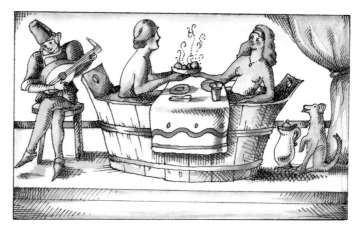

Orgies were commonplace. Musicians played while bathers sang, danced, drank, made love, and ate from floating trays. As a result of the scandals, a ban was placed on mixed bathing. The ringing of bells announced the appropriate time for each sex to bathe. The wealthy and idle still spent much of their time lavishing together in perfumed water. It was not unheard of to discover someone had died in the bath after indulging in an evening of wanton activity.

The early Christians rejected the public bath houses of Rome. Some abstained from bathing, thus mortifying the flesh as a penance for sins. A more moderate view was preached later in the Middle Ages when only cold water baths were acceptable. Private baths were the order of the day. Wooden tubs with boards placed across them for playing cards and dining were large enough to accommodate two. Even in cold water, bathing was a time for socializing.

Spiritual cleansing was practiced in the form of a quick plunge in cold water for baptism, or washing of the hands before ritual. In many cases, water became the vehicle for divine healing. Wells and streams were identified with saints who had used the water or died near the site. For a squire to become a knight, he was required to take a ritual cold bath on the eve of his knighthood. The squire was escorted by two "esquires of honor brave" to a barber who shaved him and trimmed his hair. He was then led to the bath, where he was undressed and doused with cold water. After the bath, he was met by the old knights of the court and led to the chapel where spiced wine was served and minstrals sang. The squire was attended to throughout the night until his honor was bestowed at sunrise.

Despite good intentions, the church was unable to stop the progression to steamier times. Hot water pleasures were inevitable. People got into trouble when they got into hot water.

Public baths were still considered wicked, and rightfully so. In England, the "Stews," or hot bath houses, were brothels. In 1546, Henry VIII had to close the Stews in order to halt the spread of syphilis.

Renaissance France gave us the bathtub as we know it. The shape was changed from round to oval, and it was large enough to recline in. Louis XIII developed a taste for sitting in water scented with rose petals. But his son

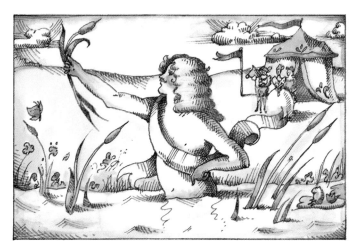

did not inherit his taste for bathing. He had the most sumptuous bathroom in Europe, but insisted on bathing only once or twice a year, in summer, in a natural spring.

Every culture has its own preference for bathing. The Russians and Swedes, living in cold climates, promote circulation by beating themselves with branches and then taking a plunge in icy water outdoors. The Japanese have raised bathing to the level of art, requiring two baths; the first for cleansing, and the second for socializing. Americans tend to prefer showers over baths. We are probably the cleanest people in the world; at least we bathe more frequently than others. Even in America, it took some time for the benefits of plumbing and advancing technology to bring the bathtub indoors. For many years, indoor bathtubs were considered unAmerican. When the first bathtub was installed in the White House in 1851, it caused an uproar. The years have proven how luxurious a bathtub in a convenient room can be. Thank goodness we have advanced. A bath is a gift for all the senses—a luxury you can afford.

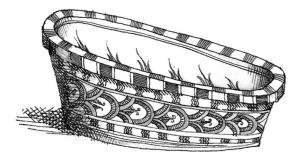

The Bathtub

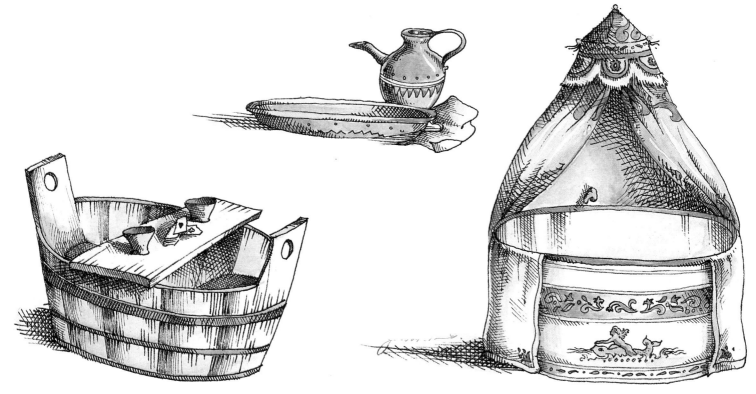

Revolutions occurred in the style and shape of bathtubs as often as they did in politics. Running outdoors for a chilly dip in a wooden tub very soon lost its romance. So man developed his intellect, and then the bathtub. As you can see, a simple bath was not always easy to find.

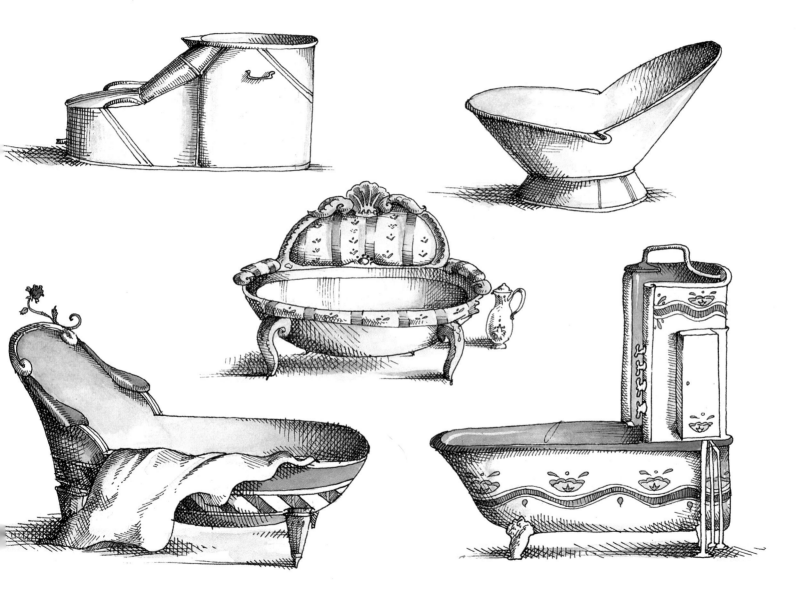

You and the Bath

I f water is the heart of a bath, then scents and fragrances are the soul. The bath is an occasion to indulge your fantasies. Now is the time to familiarize yourself with the many delightful ways you can scent your tub.

The recipes in these pages are designed to make each bath special. Some are old remedies which come from as far back as the Middle Ages. Others were passed down in my family or came from friends. I invented many of the recipes after lots and lots of baths. Most of the recipes are easy to make...and fun. You can be steeping tonight in a wonderfully fragrant bath while preparing others for tomorrow.

It takes time to create some of the ingredients for the recipes. Here is an introduction to the different types of fragrances for the bath, with instructions for preparing them. Once you know the basics, the rest will be a breeze.

Essences

Perfume contains many ingredients, but the most important is "essential oil." Essential oils are distilled from flowering plants, and retain their scent. Lighter than true oils, they do not leave a mark after evaporating. Extracting the essence from a flower is a very involved process. All of the essences required for recipes can be found in beauty shops or health food stores. For the ambitious, I have included instructions for extracting your own essences, or "Enfleurage," on pages 24 and 25.

Oils

Body and bath oils provide wonderful fragrances, but they also protect the skin. Water is the basis of young-looking skin, and oils hold moisture in. The best oils are light and easily absorbed. Mineral oil is used most often, but almond oil, olive oil, apricot oil, castor oil, coconut oil, and palm oil may be used. To infuse oil with a desired scent, follow these instructions:

2 cups oil   ¾ cup desired herb or flower, fresh or dried.

Combine ingredients, and let stand for one week in a glass jar. Strain and repeat until desired strength is achieved.

Colognes

The first cologne was discovered by a botanist in ancient times, who placed dried, scented flowers in white wine and found that the scented wine retained the perfume of the flower longer than the flower alone. Today colognes are made by combining alcohol with a few drops of essential oil and water. Several essences are usually combined to create the fragrance in a cologne. The result is a delicate scent that lingers longer than a floral or bath water, but not as long as perfume. When added to bath water, or applied after-bath, cologne leaves the skin tingling and refreshed. You can concoct your own cologne!

1½ cup alcohol   1-2 tsp. floral essence(s)   3 tsp. water

Combine ingredients, and use directly. Or store in a tightly stopped glass bottle until ready to apply.

Floral Waters

Scented water may be used directly on the skin as a refreshing splash, or may be added liberally to warm water for a subtly fragrant bath. It is easy and satisfying to make.

1 oz. essence   1 qt. distilled water

Combine ingredients and use alone, or use in other recipes for cologne, scented baths, moisturizers, etc.

Bath Vinegars

One of the most important elements of healthy skin is the acid-mantle, a chemical balance of the outer layer of the skin. Soaps and alkaline makeup can disturb the acid-mantle, causing itching and flaking. The best way to retain the proper balance is to use an astringent lotion. It may be used directly on the skin or added to bath water. Most commercial astringents contain a high percentage of alcohol, which can be drying. Vinegars are more soothing and better for the skin. You will be surprised how pleasant a delicately fragrant bath vinegar can be.

1 cup desired herb or flower   2 cups white wine vinegar

Combine ingredients and steep for 2 weeks in direct sunlight. Shake the bottle daily. For skin freshener, combine 1 part vinegar with 8 parts water. For bathing, add ¼ to ½ cup vinegar to warm bath water.

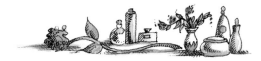

Preserving

NOTE:

It is important to be aware of the perishable properties of homemade recipes. I have included some natural preservatives such as alcohol, essential oils, and vinegar in the recipes. It is best to use fresh ingredients in small amounts, and use them immediately. When in doubt, refrigerate the mixture.

Brewing and Steeping

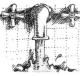

here are as many wonderful uses for herbs and teas in the tub as there are at the family table. I have found that bathing in infused water can have remarkably restorative results. Herbs and teas can be used externally as stimulants or relaxants. They can soothe the skin, help stimulate circulation, promote sleep, relieve aches in muscles and joints, or may be enjoyed as a delightful aromatic. Many of the recipes in these pages call for infusions of herbs and teas. Here is the proper way to brew them.

Pot Brewing

Herbs and teas can be brewed in a pot loosely or with a tea egg. Add the recommended amount of tea or herb to the tea egg or directly to the pot, and pour in boiling water. Let steep for 15 minutes. Strain first if brewed loosely; add directly to the bath water if brewed with a tea egg. Never brew herbs or teas in a metal container. They will take on an unpleasant flavor and scent.

Faucet Brewing

Make a bath sachet for this unique brewing process. Fill a 4-inch square of cheesecloth with ¼–½ cup herb or tea. Tie the sachet securely, and suspend it under the faucet of your bathtub. Allow the sachet to hang under fast-running bath water; the tub will fill with a marvellous fragrance. The sachet may be added to the bath water for a more potent aroma.

Commercial tea bags may be used in this manner, as can tea eggs. Be careful to attach the bags or egg securely when in use.

Herbs and Teas
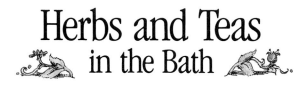 in the Bath

Anise   Stimulating, aromatic, this is a fine fragrance for men. It is made by distilling the root, seeds, or fruit of the plant. In ancient times, anise was used to pay taxes.

Basil   Relaxing, aromatic. Basil was once thought to have given witches their magical powers. In the bath, it creates a sweet, soothing effect.

Bay   Aromatic. Bay leaves come from trees of the laurel family, which were considered symbols of glory and are said to have come from the trees of Apollo. Bay is a fine blending herb.

Birch Bark   Soothing, healing. This infusion has been used since ancient times as a remedy for irritations of the skin. It is a natural astringent.

Black Tea   Soothing. All black tea contains tannin, which is a natural healing agent, and protects the skin. In the bath it is a remedy for sunburn.

Calendula   Soothing, healing. The dried flowers of this plant make an aromatic bath.

Camomile   Stimulating, healing. This herb was greatly loved by the ancient Egyptians. It is known as a symbol of ingenuity. When used in the bath, this herb soothes swelling, irritated skin, and repels insects. The powdered flowers will bring out the highlights in blonde hair; apply after shampooing and rinse out.

Cinnamon   Aromatic. The bark of the cinnamon tree, when infused in bath water, is wonderfully fragrant; it is a good blending aromatic.

Comfrey   Soothing. This herb has been used for centuries to heal bruises and other irritations of the skin when infused in bath water.

Cucumber   Soothing, cooling. This herb and its juice have been used throughout history as a beauty aid and skin freshener. It may be applied directly to skin, or added to bath water.

Dandelion   Stimulating. The leaves and root of this herb can be infused to revive skin, and is mildly astringent. It is known as a symbol of future love.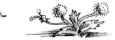

Elder Flower   Relaxing, aromatic. Elder is considered the symbol of compassion. The tree was once planted in houses to keep away witches. When used in the bath, it is a sweet-scented tonic for skin and eyes. Mildly astringent.

Geranium Root   Soothing, healing. An infusion of this herb will help heal minor irritations of the skin.

Ginger   Stimulating, aromatic. Ginger is known as an aphrodisiac, and was thought to have turned frigid women into enchantresses. When added to bath water, it promotes circulation and is warming in winter time.

Horse Chestnut   Soothing. The seed of this tree contains tannin and, when infused, makes a fine, healthy bath. Naturally astringent.

Jasmine   Aromatic. Infusion made from the tea or essential oil of this flower is wonderfully fragrant. A fine blending scent.

Juniper   Stimulating, soothing, aromatic. A bath in an infusion of juniper berries or shoots is good for aching joints or muscles.

Kelp   Refreshing. This plant grows in huge oceanic forests and, when added to bath water or sachet, can be restorative to skin.

Lavender   Relaxing, healing, aromatic. The fragrant flowers of this plant have been used for centuries in perfumes and cleansers. The word comes from the Latin *lavare* — to wash. It is fine alone or when mixed with other herbs and fragrances.

Lemon   Cleansing. Lemon is the symbol of harvest. A natural astringent, it is aromatic and freshening when used in the bath.

Lemon Grass   Refreshing. This herb can be fragrant and cooling in summer baths.

Linden   Soothing. This herb is fine for soothing frayed nerves, when infused in bath water.

Mint   Stimulant, soothing. This wonderfully fragrant herb is known for being an aphrodisiac, and a symbol of abandonment. It makes a great cooling and toning bath.

Nettle   Healing. This plant has been used throughout history for its healing properties. It leaves hair shining when used as a rinse.

Orange   Aromatic. Makes a fine blending fragrance.

Parsley   Stimulant. This herb was valued by the ancient Romans as a tonic for the skin. It is mildly aromatic.

Peppermint   Stimulant. This is a symbol of friendship. It is soothing, and a natural antiseptic.

Pine   Stimulant. This will make a fragrant and toning bath, as well as being a fine air freshener. Naturally antiseptic.

Rose   Relaxing, soothing, aromatic. This is the favorite fragrance around the world, and a symbol of Love. It is revitalizing when used in the bath. Slightly astringent.

Rosemary   Stimulating, soothing. This therapeutic herb is known as a symbol of loyalty and remembrance. It will soothe nerves when bathed in, and makes a wonderful hair rinse for brunettes.

Sage   Stimulant. Sage is a symbol of virtue. It is naturally astringent and deodorant. May be used as a rinse for covering gray hair.

Soapwort   Bubbling. The leaves and the pink and white flowers of this herb foam when bruised and added to bath water.

Spearmint   Soothing. This will make a fragrant and tonic bath for the skin.

Thyme   Stimulating. Known as the love herb, thyme is a muscle relaxant and will soothe cramps and aching joints when infused in bath water. Natural astringent.

Vanilla Grass   Aromatic. Strewn in the doorways of Russian churches, this herb has a delicate, sweet scent and is wonderful in the bath.

Walnut Leaf   Soothing. A bath from these leaves will promote sleep and soothe nerves.

Yarrow   Relaxing. The ancient Chinese valued this herb. It is a natural astringent, and soothes muscle aches when infused in bath water.

For Your Tub

 bath should begin in a cheery room; clean, light, and warm. Scents are heavenly for nose and nerves, but to step out really refreshed, you must stock your tub with the right accessories, too.

Bath sponges come in all shapes, sizes, and textures. They stimulate circulation while drenching the skin with moisture. Scrubbers also come in many forms. The loofah is a natural fiber scrub, and is said to aid in the elimination of cellulite. I am not sure if this is true, but it gives a wonderful friction rub for rough skin and aching muscles. Brushes will help circulation, too, and rid skin of older surface cells which can leave skin feeling flaky. Hand mitts and towels serve the same purpose.

Bath trays and baskets are a must. They are handy for holding scrubs, soap, toys, etc. Some dangle from the shower head, others span the tub and allow you to eat or write or read while reclining.

Treat yourself to some of the remarkable bath toys available. Diving fish and boats, puzzles, balls, books, and, of course, rubber ducks will amuse you while you bathe.

Hand-held shower attachments deserve special mention. They are a revolution in bath technology. Most models come with a massage adjustment. Once you become accustomed to a massage while bathing, you cannot imagine doing without. Hand-held attachments are also great for washing and rinsing hair. Best of all, I've found they make cleaning the tub a breeze.

The more choices you have for a bath, the better. Continue adding to your collection!

16

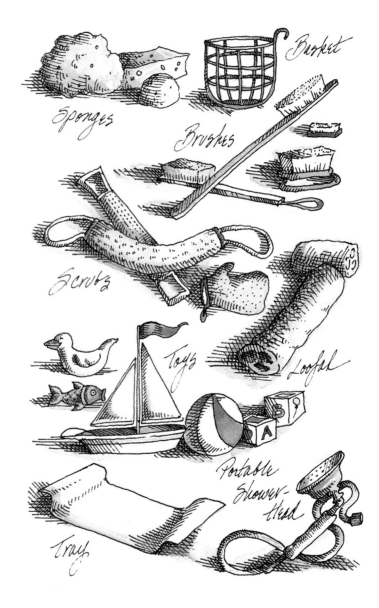

Sponges

Basket

Brushes

Scrubs

Loofah

Toys

Portable Shower-Head

Tray

Bottles and Boxes

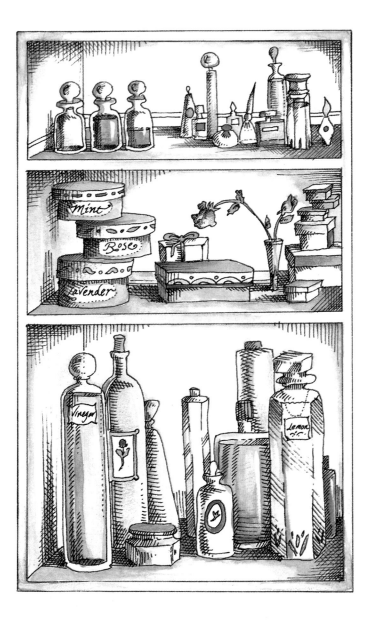

our dressing table is an important part of the bath. Now is the time to appoint it with beautiful containers for your bath recipes. Imagine how delightful it will be to select your fragrances from a variety of vials. How charming to dust yourself with sweetly scented powder from a paisleyed box. These containers must be functional as well as pleasing to the eye. Glass jars and bottles must be tightly stopped, and boxes must be lined for freshness.

Start by spending an afternoon at your community flea market or swap meet. I've found all sorts of bottles, jars, and boxes there. If you select carefully, you can find little treasures, usually for a song. Department stores and boutiques sell lovely copies of antique perfume bottles. If you really want to splurge, find your way to an antique shop. They sell gorgeous bottles from the turn of the century and earlier. These bottles are often made of cut crystal with elegantly etched designs and labels. They will not come cheap but you will enjoy them each time you use them.

Look for boxes with tight-fitting lids. Keep them lined with linen or cheesecloth. This helps keep the moisture out, and will help preserve your dried herbs and flowers. Cover boxes with exotic papers from Italy or Japan, or with silk. Make your own painted labels, with designs or pictures of herbs. If you keep powders in boxes, you can find dusting puffs sold individually at most pharmacies. A trick I discovered is to keep bath powder in an antique salt shaker, which can be handily sprinkled after bath.

I suggest a mix of jars and boxes. Design your dressing table to your own needs and taste. Enjoy!

Soap and Shampoo

oap is the oldest cleanser in the world. It was first used 2,300 years ago by the Phoenecians who mixed goat's tallow with beech ashes. It was so harsh that it burned the skin. Centuries later, gentle soaps were invented. The first soap makers in Europe appeared in England in the 12th century. But soap was a luxury. Common people almost never were able to afford it, and the wealthy preferred not to use it. In 1672, a German gentleman sent his lady a beautiful treasure box filled with soap worth its weight in gold. It was necessary to include detailed instructions on its use. This aversion to soap and bathing may account for the rise in popularity of perfume in Europe. People did not use soap regularly for cleansing until the Industrial Revolution, when it became possible to manufacture soap on a mass scale. Before that, people in America and Europe made soap at home. Here is the basic recipe for home-made soap.

4 oz. lye   10 oz. water

24 oz. tallow

Recipe makes 2.3 pounds of soap. You'll need 2 stainless steel meat thermometers, one for the lye solution and one for the fat solution. Wearing rubber gloves, carefully mix water with lye. Note the rising temperature (due to the chemical reaction between lye and water). Allow to cool. Melt fat over low heat, and place the pot in a pan of cold water. While fat temperature cools to 120-130°, place lye solution in a pan of warm water. When lye solution cools to 85-95°, carefully combine lye and fat, mixing slowly. Stir constantly until mixture reaches the consistency of honey. Pour mixture into molds or tin boxes lined with wax paper. Set overnight wrapped in a blanket or towel. Let unmolded cakes age 2 weeks before using. If fragrant soap is desired, add ¼ oz. of essential oil of your choice to fat when melting.

Soaps and shampoos come in hundreds of colors, textures, and fragrances, but they are all designed to clean. Most commercial products contain ingredients that promote their ability to bubble. And although they are safe, they can sometimes disturb the sensitive chemical balance of skin and scalp. I suggest a wash or rinse with an astringent mixture every 2 weeks. This will keep hair shining and scalp healthy.

Egg Hair Rinse

2 beaten eggs   1 tsp. lemon juice

Whisk ingredients and work into wet hair. Leave for 5 mintues and then rinse with warm water.

Champagne Hair Rinse

1 cup champagne

Rinse through hair after cleansing, and allow to set for 5 mintues. Rinse thoroughly. Will leave hair conditioned without an unpleasant odor.

Lemon Hair Rinse

juice of 2 lemons   ½ cup hot water

Combine the juice of the lemons with the hot water and rinse through hair after cleansing. Leaves hair shining, and promotes highlights.

Raspberry Vinegar Wash

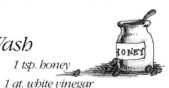

½ cup raspberries   1 tsp. honey

½ tsp. crushed cloves   1 qt. white vinegar

Combine ingredients and set for 1 week, shaking the bottle daily. Mix 1 part vinegar to 6 parts water. Rinse through hair after cleansing. Leaves hair squeaky clean and scalp soothed.

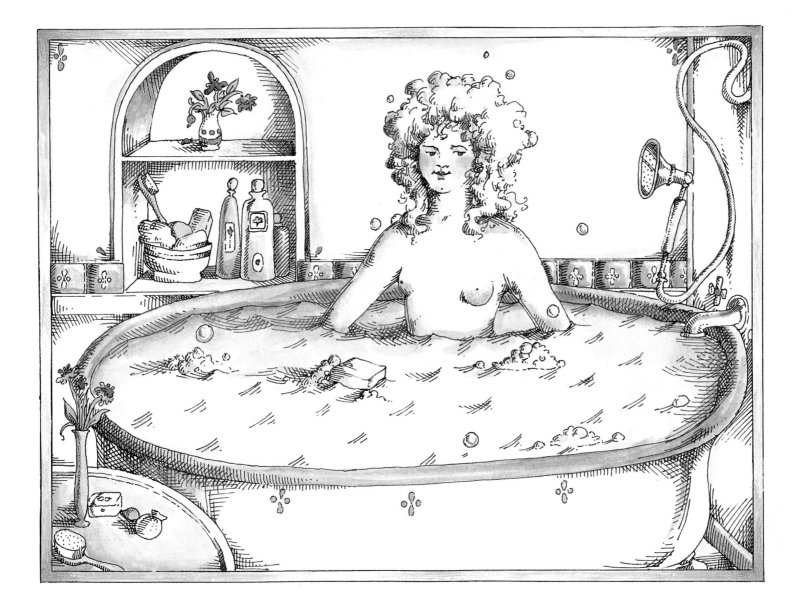

Things You'll Need

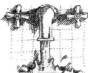

he kitchen is the place to begin thinking about preparing recipes for the bath. Many of the items you will be using are already on your cupboard shelves.

Commercial herbs and spices may be used for the recipes. But if you have an herb garden, use fresh herbs, or dry them for later baths.

Utensils are basic. Brewing pots should be made of glass, china, or porcelain. If herbs are brewed in a metal vessel, the infusion will take on an unpleasant flavor and scent. All utensils should be kept clean and dry. I collect and use old jam jars and wine bottles for steeping recipes. You will need one or two large vessels for this purpose. Clean glass jars carefully. Any traces of previous contents will spoil the delicate scents of these recipes.

A place should be made in the kitchen to house dried herbs and flower petals. The pantry is the best place for storage, but any cool, dry, fairly dark corner will do. Keep dried herbs and flowers in tightly-stopped jars or boxes.

Clean utensils with a little baking soda and vinegar. Besides being effective cleansers, they are economical, safe, and will not spoil a concoction if residue remains.

Most recipes in these pages can be made easily and quickly. Take time to read a recipe before-hand so you will have time to acquire any ingredients or utensils you may need.

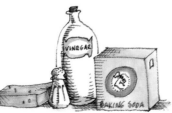

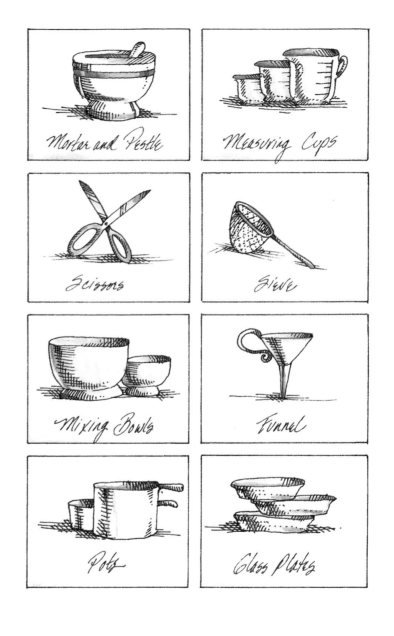

Mortar and Pestle

Measuring Cups

Scissors

Sieve

Mixing Bowls

Funnel

Pots

Glass Plates

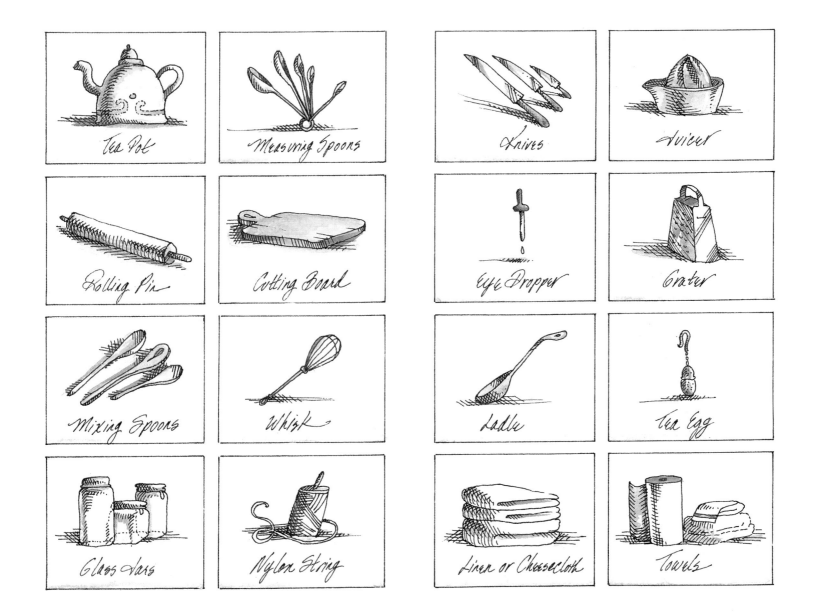

Tea Pot

Measuring Spoons

Knives

Juicer

Rolling Pin

Cutting Board

Eye Dropper

Grater

Mixing Spoons

Whisk

Ladle

Tea Egg

Glass Jars

Nylon String

Linen or Cheesecloth

Towels

The Spring Bath

Renewal! The air is light and the sun is high in the sky. Green shoots are beginning to break ground in the garden. Romance! The checkout boy at the market becomes strangely alluring. You have impulses to take long walks in the middle of a sales strategy meeting. If only you could get home to a luxurious bath.

Springtime bathing is probably the most romantic and pleasurable of all. Perfumes and scents are made from the blossoms of springtime flowers. This is the time to collect and dry flower petals for the sachets, oils and essences you will use year 'round. Use your bathtub as an instrument of love, or as a haven for simple, blissful privacy.

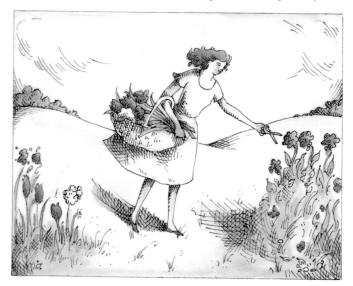

The Lavender Bath

Lavender may be used to encourage sleep. It is a relaxing, fragrant bath.

1 oz. dried lavender   *½ oz. rosemary*

2 cups white vinegar

Combine ingredients and let stand one week. Shake the jar daily. Add ¼ to ½ cup to bath water, or mix 1 part vinegar to 8 parts water for a refreshing, astringent splash.

The French Beauty Bath Sachet

Nino de Lenclos, a famous beauty of the old French court, used this recipe to retain her youthful appearance. It worked so well that her grandson fell in love with her, having never seen her before. The romance was cut short when the true nature of their relationship was discovered.

One handful of each: lavender   *rosemary*   *2 cups water*

mint   *thyme*

Mix in a linen or cheesecloth square, tie, and steep in boiling water for 10 minutes, or brew under fast-running bath water.

The Peppermint Bath

Beside refreshing and invigorating, this bath can sooth aching joints or strained muscles.

½ cup fresh peppermint leaves

½ cup juniper berries or shoots

1 qt. water

Steep leaves and berries in boiling water for 10 minutes, strain, and add to warm bath water.

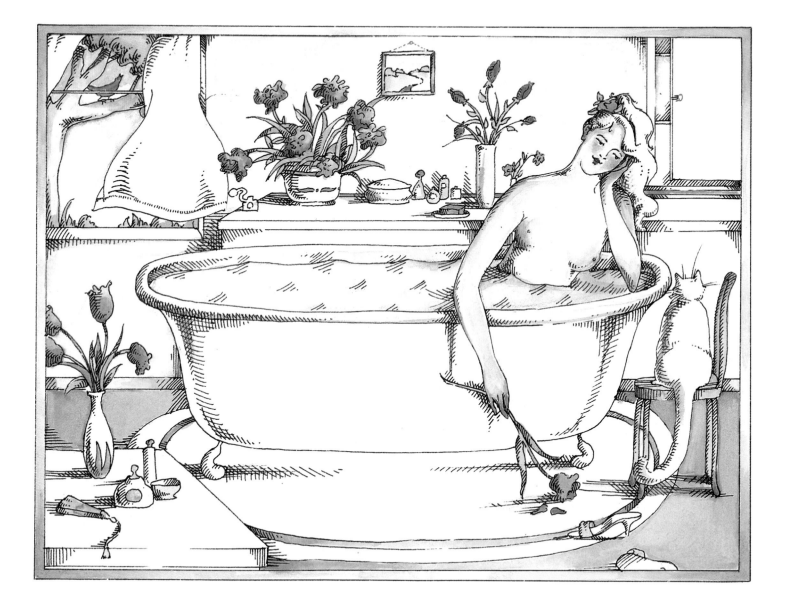

Enfleurage

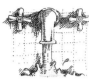hroughout the ages women have dabbed the essence of rose, jasmine, lavender, and gardenia behind their ears and at their breasts to attract the object of their desires. The essence of flowers are the oldest perfumes, used since the time of Nefertiti to attract and entice. Cleopatra used perfume to attract Julius Caesar and Mark Antony. Queen Elizabeth I was an amateur perfumer and went so far as to require the ladies of her court to keep perfumed boxes, or "scented coffer," at their bedsides. Madame Pompadour sent a special guard of Louis XV's army around the world to gather the flowers and herbs she desired for her scented baths. Catherine the Great of Russia once kept an ambassador waiting while she languished in a floral bath, and almost caused an international incident. Be assured, the essences of flowers are powerful and alluring. No woman should be without her own special scent.

The French word for extracting the scent from flowers is "enfleurage." Rose and violet are the oldest scents, but jasmine, hyacinth, lily of the valley, lilac, mock orange, gardenia, and magnolia have wonderful bouquets, too.

During the process, petals are spread upon glass plates which have been coated with fat. Over time, this fat is saturated with the scent of the petals. It is then dissolved and mixed with other ingredients to become perfume.

For those of you with time on your hands, or if you are adventuresome, try making your own essences. They can be made at home with patience and care. Most essence can be found in stores, and are much easier to buy than make. If you're a purist, however, this is the way to go.

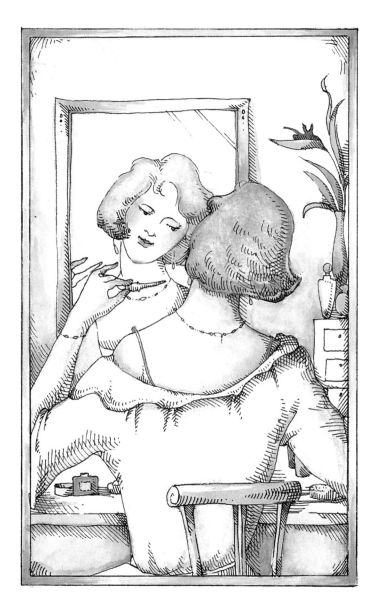

Classic Enfleurage

Utensils: 2 glass pie plates

1 quart jar with screw lid   2 12-inch muslin squares

Ingredients: ¾ pound animal fat or Crisco

¼ lb. lard   1 qt. distilled water

1 tsp. alum   1 pt. alcohol

1 pt. white wine

Fresh flower petals—Approx. ½ cup every 3 days for 1 month
Total: 7½ cups

Combine fat, lard, water, and alum and bring to a boil. Alum is the root of the geranium, and is used here in a dried, powdered form. It is an astringent and may be found in health food or herbalist shops.

When fat is dissolved, strain through one of the muslin cloths, and discard the cloth. Reheat the remaining liquid and then pour into the 2 glass pie plates. Allow to cool. Drain off any remaining water.

Sprinkle fresh flower petals over the surface of one filled glass dish. Add petals to 1-inch thickness. Invert the second dish over the first, and leave undisturbed for 2–3 days.

Continue adding fresh petals every 2–3 days until blooming season ends, or for 1 month. By this time the fat has absorbed the scent of the petals.

Place the mixture in the glass jar, adding equal parts of wine and alcohol. Place the jar in a dark closet for 2–3 months, shaking the bottle daily.

Now strain the liquid through the second muslin cloth, and use to scent bath water and cologne, or as perfume.

Salt Enfleurage

Utensils: Mortar and pestle   1 pint jar with lid

Ingredients: ¼ cup table salt   1 cup fresh rose petals

1 gal. distilled water

Bruise the petals in the mortar and pestle. Mix the salt together with the bruised petals and place in the jar. Add 2 or 3 teaspoons of the mixture to 1 gallon of distilled water to make rose water.

Quick Classic Enfleurage

Utensils: 1 glass pie plate

3 or 4 muslin squares cut to fit the pie plate

Ingredients: ½ cup mineral oil

Fresh flower petals—Approx. 1½ cups every 2 days for 2 weeks
Total: 10½ cups

Fill the pie plate 1-inch deep with fresh flower petals. Soak the muslin cloths in oil, and place one of them over the flower petals. Continue layering petals and cloths until the stack is several inches high. Leave undisturbed for 2 days, then replace the flower petals. When the cloths are sufficiently saturated with the flower perfume (about 2 weeks), press oil from the cloths into a bottle. Use as you would any floral essence.

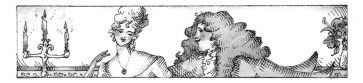

Water Enfleurage

Utensils: 1 glass pie plate

1 small glass jar with screw lid

Ingredients: 1 cup rain water

Fresh flower petals–Approx. ½ cup every 2 days for 2 weeks
Total: 3½ cups

Place the glass pie plate filled with water in direct sunlight. Cover the water's surface with a ¼-inch layer of flower petals. Leave undisturbed for 2 days. Be sure to use enough water to allow for evaporation. After 2 days, a film should appear on the surface fo the water. This contains the essential oil of the flower. Continue adding flower petals and small amounts of water for 2 weeks. When ready, skim the film from the surface of the water and place it in the small bottle. Let any water evaporate before capping the bottle. Use the essence to scent cupboards, drawers, or sachets for the bath.

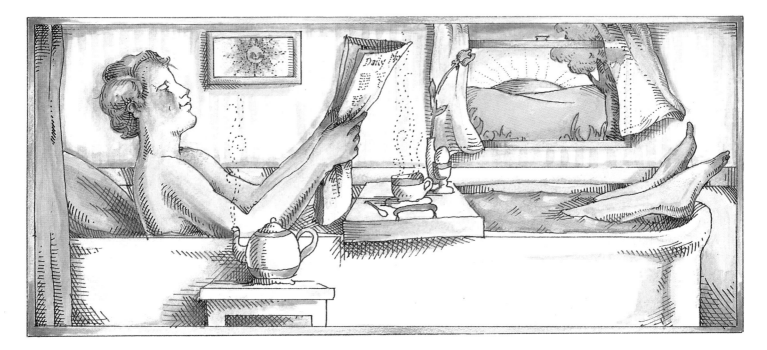

The Sunrise Bath

The sun is up, the birds are chattering. Rise and greet the day with a pleasing soak. Give yourself some time to collect your thoughts, even if it means setting the alarm early.

Enjoy a light repast. My feeling about eating in the tub is, if it can survive getting wet and still be delectable, it's appropriate. I suggest fresh berries or melon, orange juice and coffee. Don't stuff yourself. Soothing bath water and a big breakfast will just put you back to sleep.

You want stimulation. Have a friction rub with a loofah or brush to get your circulation going.

If you exercise in the morning, a bath will be just the thing to help you gather your thoughts before setting off into the day. Many people shower after a morning jog, but a bath can be just as stimulating, and more soothing. Morning baths should be long enough to revive and cleanse. Keep the bath water on the cool side; at about 80-90°. This will act as a tonic. Try a quick, cool-water sponge rinse before rising from the tub. It will close your pores and reduce your chance of catching a chill.

Aromatic Sage Bath

Sage is a stimulating herb, as well as being a natural deodorant.

1 oz. dried sage	*½ oz. lavender*
½ oz. rosemary	*2 ½ cups water*

Steep ingredients in boiling water for 10 minutes and add to bath water. Finish with a light sprinkle of scented bath powder.

Eucalyptus Bath

Eucalyptus is warming and stimulating, and will help open sleepy eyes. It will fill the room with a superb fragrance.

2 tsp. eucalyptus oil

Make scented oil as per instructions on page 13, using fresh eucalyptus cuttings. Add oil to fast-running bath water.

Dawn Bath

Lovage is naturally deodorizing, and makes a refreshing morning bath.

1 oz. lovage root   *1 pinch lavender*

1½ cups water

Steep lovage and lavendar in boiling water for 10–15 minutes, strain, and add to bath water.

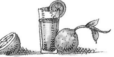

Orange Bath

Sip some orange juice along with this bath. It is a sweet way to begin the day.

1½ oz. essence of orange or mock orange

1 gallon distilled water

Mix and add liberally to bath water for a fragrant morning soak.

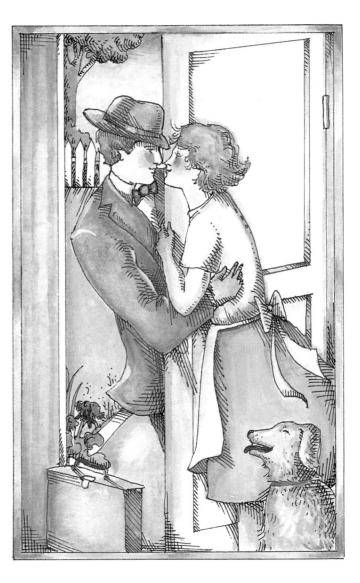

The Summer Bath

few years ago, after a particularly long and rainy spring, I awoke to a glorious summer morning. The sun was bright, and the air was so sweet that I grabbed a towel and headed for the seashore. I bared my limbs to the sun, ran into the surf, and basked for hours on the warm sand. Meanwhile, my winter pallor turned lobster red.

That night my skin was scorched, and I was barely able to move. My Great Aunt Celia (who claims to have had a premonition of my sorry state) telephoned just in the nick of time from Atlanta. As soon as she heard my voice and verified my condition, she issued me this order: "Catherine darlin', go to the kitchen this minute and put the kettle on. I want you to brew the strongest, blackest pot of Darjeeling tea you can, and pour it into a tub full of water. Then sit there for a good long time. Don't you wait another minute, honey . . . you call me in the mornin', hear?"

I never found out whether Southern girls were the first to know the secret of black tea baths, but Great Aunt Celia did. Tannin found in black tea and coffee is a remedy for burns, and promotes the tanning rather than reddening of over-exposed skin. My sunburn healed more comfortably and quickly than ever before, and Great Aunt Celia received a large tin of Darjeeling tea for her trouble.

My foolishness taught me a lesson. Now I bask in moderation; before or after noon when the sun's rays are least damaging, and I always wear a moisturizing sun screen.

Don't make a habit of overexposing your skin, but if you find yourself in a similar predicament, try one of these soothing baths.

28

Aunt Celia's Sun Bath

When added to bath water, black tea will promote browning of sunburned skin.

1 oz. black tea (any type)   2 cups water

Make a bath sachet, or fill a tea egg with tea. Brew in boiling water, or suspend under running bath water for 15 minutes.

Tender Cider Bath

Cider vinegar added to bath water will soothe irritated skin. It is best to bathe in a vinegar bath a day or two after sunning, when the skin has browned. It will return the skin to its normal ph balance and will relieve itching and peeling.

½ cup cider vinegar

Add vinegar to warm bath water.

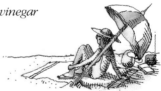

Soda Bath

Baking soda is an all-season bath ingredient, but is very soothing to sunburned skin. It is also helpful in soothing insect bites, and should be kept on-hand all summer long.

¼–½ cup baking soda

Add soda to bath water. Use more if desired.

Gentle Flower Bath

Camomile has been used since ancient times to soothe irritated skin. It brings down swelling and lightens the skin.

3–4 oz. dried camomile flowers   1 qt. water

Steep flowers in boiling water for 1 hour, strain and add to warm bath water.

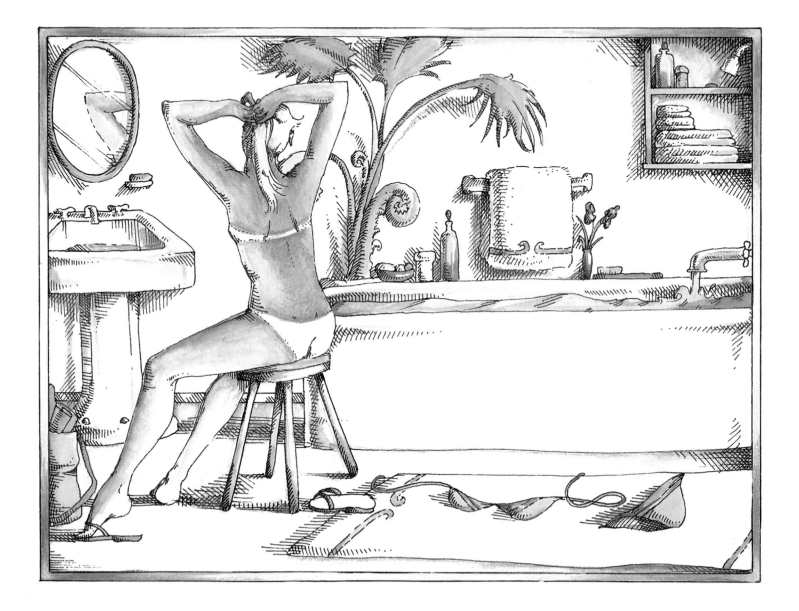

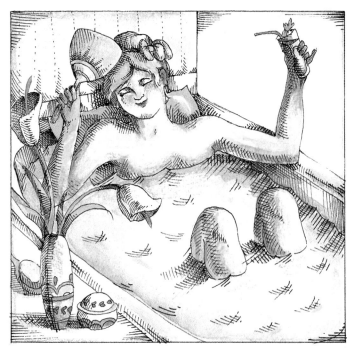

Cooling Baths

For cooling down on hot summer afternoons, try bathing in cool water (75–85°). Allow yourself some time to soak, and sip your favorite icy beverage. You'll find, as your body temperature lowers, adding warm water to the tub will be more comfortable. This makes the air temperature feel cooler after bath. Dim the room, fill a vase with summer flowers, and put your favorite music on the stereo. (A Bosanova is my favorite on hot days.) Try one or two of these recipes for a fragrant solution to the summer heat.

Mint Bath

When added to bath water, mint is wonderfully cooling in summer.

2 oz. crushed mint leaves (fresh)   2 cups water

Make a sachet or fill a tea egg with the mint leaves. Brew under running bath water, or steep in boiling water, for 15 minutes.

Lemon Mint Bath

This is one of the most refreshing baths you can indulge in on a hot summer afternoon.

1 cup fresh lemon juice   ¹/₂ cup fresh mint leaves

2 tsp. almond oil

Steep crushed mint leaves in lemon juice overnight in the refrigerator. Strain, and add almond oil. Pour under fast-running bath water for a delightful and cleansing bath. If you like, add a teaspoon or two of lemon-mint juice to a glass of iced water and sip while you soak.

Marigold Bath

Marigold is a natural healing remedy, and will soothe exposed summer skin. Camomile is soothing and will repel biting insects, too.

1¹/₂ oz. marigold flowers   1 tsp. lavender   2 cups water

1 tsp. rose petals   1 tsp. camomile

Make a bath sachet of the herbs, and steep in boiling water for 15 mintues. Add to bath water.

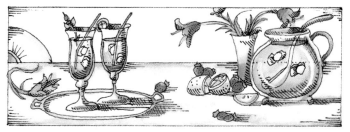

Outdoor Bathing

Swimming in the sea, lakes, rivers, and streams is a special summer pleasure. There is nothing more invigorating than a dip in the waves or languishing at your favorite swimming hole. But take proper precautions.

Always be aware of the condition of the water before entering for a swim. Currents and undertows are not always visible on the surface of the water. Never swim alone, always take along a friend. And, just as your mother said, wait a few minutes after eating before you swim.

Be especially mindful of water temperature in spas and hot tubs. It is easy for your body to feel adjusted to temperatures which are too high. Lingering in hot water can be dangerous for the elderly, or for people with heart conditions or circulatory problems. Water temperature of around 95–105° is best. The warmer the water, the shorter the soak should be. Be sure to keep water clean and chlorinated.

Summer is the most important time of year to protect your skin. Sun-screens are a must, and should be applied every time you go out in the sun. Consult your doctor for the proper number protection, and apply it at least ½ hour before exposing your skin to the sun. A sun-screen works best when applied in the shade, but must be re-applied after swimming or heavy perspiring. Begin to use it on the very first day of summer.

After bathing in sun and sea, apply a moisturizing lotion. Continue to use a moisturizer for several days following your day in the sun. If you find yourself peeling, use a gentle brush while bathing. Your tan will be the envy of everyone you meet!

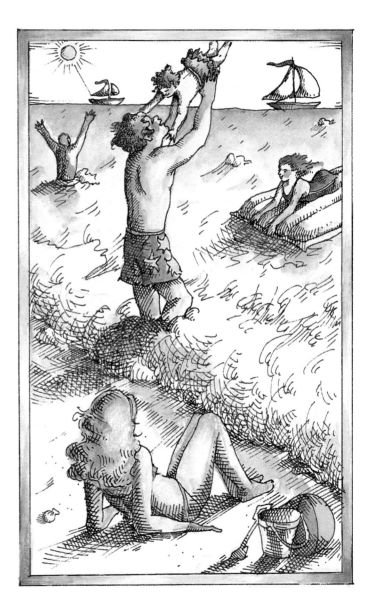

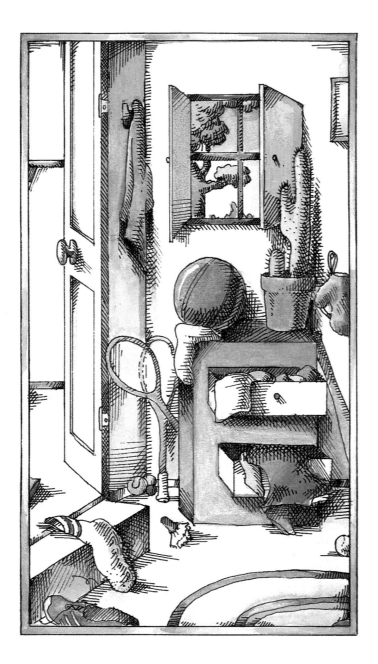

The Sports Bath

No pain, no gain? Even the most accomplished tennis, hockey, football, basketball, water-polo, or ping-pong player can pull a muscle.

It's Friday night ... your neighbor challenges you to a three-hour racquet ball game. Saturday a.m. ... it's a five mile jog around the park ... Saturday p.m., your weekly softball game. Sunday ... you take a 20 mile bike ride, and by sundown, you're a mass of aching muscles. Weekends are spent getting into shape, weekdays are spent recovering. It's a familiar story.

It is easy to overdo it. Some pain goes with the territory, too much indicates a problem. Listen to your body. It will tell you when it's had enough.

Help ease the sting of overexertion with a soothing bath and body rub. Warm water and a gentle massage can do wonders. Don't be timid about giving yourself a massage. You can tend to feet, legs, arms, torso, head, neck, and shoulders yourself. (Ask someone special to do your back.) Bath creams can be worked into aching muscles right in the tub, relieving tension while nourishing the skin. It won't make you a better hitter, but you'll feel considerably more comfortable.

Silver Birch Bath

Birch bark is an ancient remedy for soothing aches in muscles and joints. It may be used after exercising, or for the discomforts of arthritis.

4 or 5 handfuls of silver birch bark   1 qt. water

Steep the bark in warm water for ½ hour. Heat for comfort and strain before adding to warm bath water. Makes a fine foot bath as well.

Juniper Bath

Juniper berries and shoots, when infused in bath water, can relieve aching joints.

½ lb. juniper berries and/or fresh roots   1 qt. water

Combine ingredients and boil for 10 minutes. Strain, and add to warm bath water.

Athlete's Rubbing Water

It is important to massage and stretch muscles which are exercised and overworked. The rubbing water makes massage easier, and can be applied after exercising or after bath.

¼ cup witchhazel   6 oz. rose water

1 tsp. violet oil

Combine and let stand for one week in a cool, dark spot. Shake the bottle daily. Use directly on the skin and massage vigorously into sore muscles.

Menthol Bath Cream

This stimulating and fragrant cream can be massaged into aching muscles directly in the tub. It is soothing and warming.

2 tsp. lanolin   1 tsp. honey

3 oz. witchhazel   3 tsp. menthol

Beat ingredients over a double boiler until creamy. Allow to cool. Refrigerate in a glass jar until ready to use.

Linseed Rubbing Water

Linseed oil is used in a variety of soaps and creams to sooth the skin. Rub this solution directly into the skin while bathing for extra special relief for aching muscles.

¼ cup linseed oil   ¼ cup water

2 Tbsp. witch-hazel

Combine and massage directly into sore muscles after exercising or in the tub.

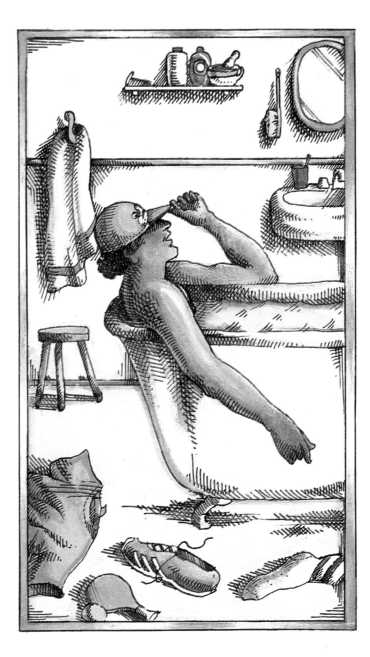

The Reflective Bath

 here are times when a bath is serious. James and I meet every Thursday for lunch downtown. By the end of the week there is lots of news, and we love to linger over every detail. It is our favorite time to visit. One day James called early on Thursday. His voice sounded tense. "Cath...I can't make it for lunch today, can you meet me for dinner?" "Sure, but what's wrong?" I asked. "It's nothing to worry about, I'll tell you all about it tonight."

That evening I put on my best dress, high heels and James' favorite perfume and drove to the restaurant expecting to find him a wreck. I ordered a bottle of his favorite champagne and waited. He arrived in a few minutes, looking radiant. I hadn't seen him look so well in ages. "What happened?...How can a person sound so miserable and then turn up looking like this?" "I have a secret. This morning Carter came in with a huge stack of files and told me to get through them by tomorrow noon. I took one look at them and my head began to throb. There's no point in our meeting when I'm in such a rotten mood. So, instead I went home and spent lunch in a nice quiet bath." "How amazing" I said. The waiter arrived with the Laurent Perrier and filled our glasses. "Not really...I've done it once or twice before, and it works every time. When I returned to the office, the work flew by. Now I'm in the right frame of mind to be with you."

Finding the time during a hectic day for a quiet bath is good for you. When you're tense and achy, you're no good to anyone, so shut the door, fill the tub with plenty of hot water, and spend an hour alone.

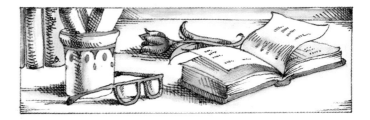

Tim's Hangover Bath

My friend Tim is a newspaper editor, and knows what a headache is all about. He says this bath works for migraines and hangovers, too.

1 cup ice cubes   1 plastic bag

small bath towel

Fill the tub with hot water. Place the ice cubes in the plastic bag, and wrap it in the bath towel. Place the ice bag at the back of your neck while reclining in the hot water. He recommends playing Handel's Messiah on the stereo as well.

Balm Bath

When infused in bath water, balm leaves are soothing and promote a gentle sleep. It is a calming bath.

2 oz. balm leaves   1 qt. water

Steep the leaves in boiling water for 10 minutes, strain, and add to warm bath water.

Soothing Lavender Bath

Lavender and basil are relaxing when added to warm bath water. The cinnamon will fill the room with a delightful aroma.

½ oz. dried lavender flowers   ½ oz. basil

1 tsp. cinnamon   1 pt. witch-hazel

Make a powder of the herbs in a mortar and pestle. Steep them in the witch-hazel for 2 weeks. Strain and add to warm bath water as desired. May be used as an after bath splash too.

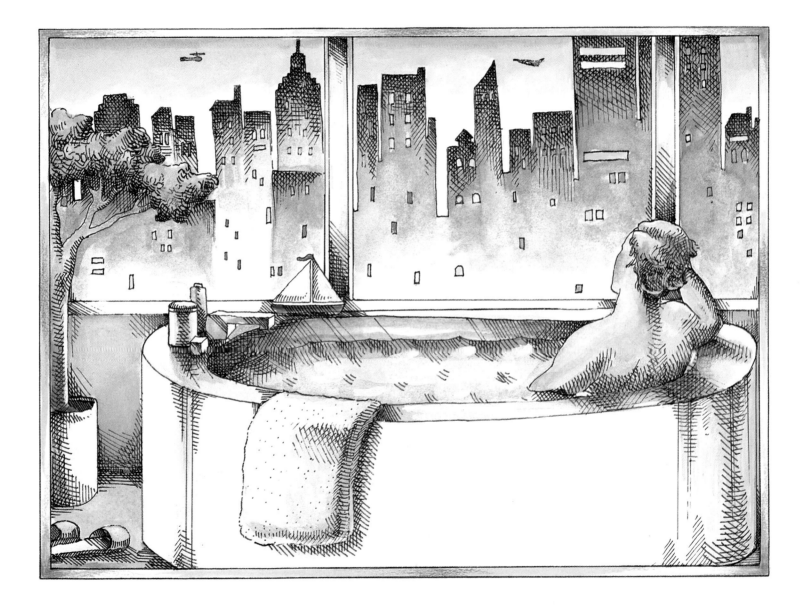

If you think the only time for a soothing bath is before bed, you're not trying. Follow my friend James' example and take your lunch break at home in the tub. How about indulging in a peaceful soak after sending the kids off to school, or steeping for an hour or so before they come home? For those of you who work full time, try a bath immediately upon arriving home. It makes a nice bridge between the hectic work day and the domestic front. It's well worth postponing dinner. You'll be less likely to burn the string beans, and you'll be a livelier conversationalist. If you have trouble sleeping, a late night bath will sooth frazzled nerves and slow you down so that you fall right to sleep.

Close your eyes. Listen to the sound of the water. Silence is a luxury. Enjoy it. Slices of cucumber can be placed on the eyelids to cool the face, and soothe strained eyes. A bath pillow at the head will ease tensions. Lower the lights and breathe deeply. Let your mind wander.

Keep simple tensions and pressures under control by enjoying a quiet bath any time. You'll feel better for it.

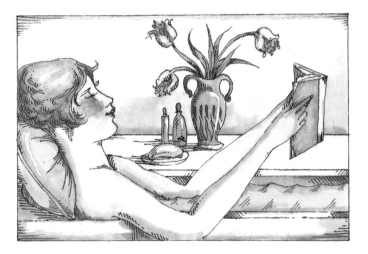

Camomile Refresher

Use this mixture directly on skin for a refreshing splash, or add to bath water for a fragrant soak.

3 to 4 oz. camomile   *1 oz. rose petals*

½ cup witchhazel   *¼ cup alcohol*

1 qt. boiling water

Steep flowers in boiling water for 1 hour. Strain, and add the alcohol and witchhazel.

Bath Thyme

Thyme in the bath will sooth and soften skin while calming your nerves.

2 tsp. dried thyme leaves and flowers   *1 tsp. fresh thyme*

1 pt. water

Steep dry and fresh thyme in boiling water for 30 minutes. Strain and add to bath water. For an extra peaceful bath, you may soak cotton balls in the infusion and cover your eyelids while bathing.

Elder Flower Milk Bath

Elder flowers in the bath will create a gentle, sweet scented soak which will revive your spirit and refresh your skin.

½ cup elder flowers   *1 pt. milk*

Soak the flowers in the milk for 3 hours. Then warm gently, strain, and add to bath water. Rose petals may be added to the milk if a more fragrant bath is desired.

Lion's Tooth Bath

This dandelion bath is refreshing and soothing to skin and nerves. Dandelion gets its name from the French "Dent-de-Lion," or lion's tooth, for the shape of the leaves.

½ lb. dandelion leaves or root   *1 qt. water*

Combine ingredients and boil. Let steep for 10 minutes, strain, and add to warm bath water.

The Spearmint Bath

Spearmint is both soothing and tonic for body and soul. Enjoy this bath in the morning for a refreshing start to the day.

½ cup spearmint water   *2 tsp. almond oil*

3 tsp. witchhazel

Make spearmint water by infusing leaves in boiling water. Combine ingredients and apply to skin while bathing. Pour remaining liquid directly into warm bath water.

Bay Leaf Bath

This is a mild and fragrant bath. Very refreshing to skin, and can be enjoyed anytime.

1 oz. bay leaves   *½ oz. mint*

½ oz. lemon grass   *½ oz. comfrey*

1½ pint vinegar

Over a low flame, heat the vinegar. Remove from heat and add the herbs. Place in direct sunlight in a glass jar for 2 weeks. Shake the jar daily. Add ½ cup to bath water, or mix 1 part vinegar to 8 parts water for an astringent lotion.

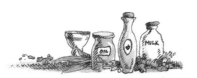

Tonic Bran Bath

This is a soothing and wonderfully aromatic bath. It smells warm and wheaty, and is very good for the skin.

½ lb. wheat bran   *½ lb. rye bran*

2 qts. water

Combine ingredients and bring to boil. Steep for 10-15 minutes, strain, and add to warm bath water.

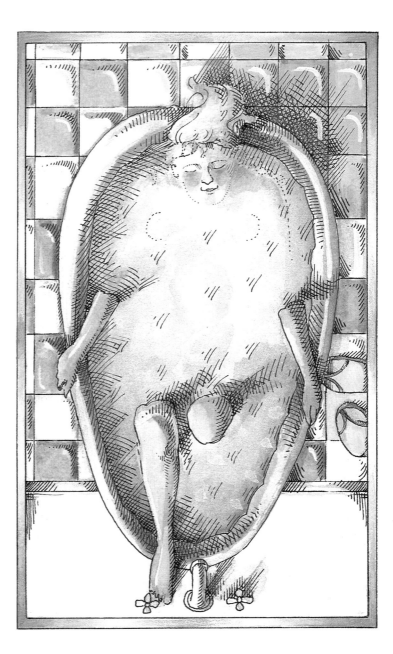

The Love Bath

bath is the perfect place for lovers: private, sensual, and warm. Kisses have been exchanged in steaming tubs for centuries. In Rome, Nero and his concubines made the shared bath infamous. During the Middle Ages, lovers bathed outdoors surrounded by minstrels, with servants providing food and wine. In the Renaissance, bathtubs were designed especially for two, with embroidered drapery for privacy, and a tray that could be placed across the tub for playing cards and dining. Casanova was known to be a great admirer of the shared bath. He described a particularly pleasant experience in a London bath house this way . . . "It makes a magnificent debauch and costs only six guineas. The cost may be cut to one hundred francs, but economy in pleasure is not to my liking."

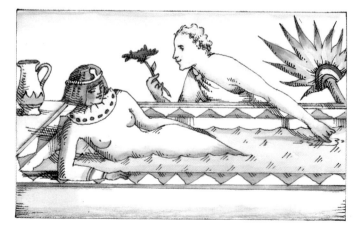

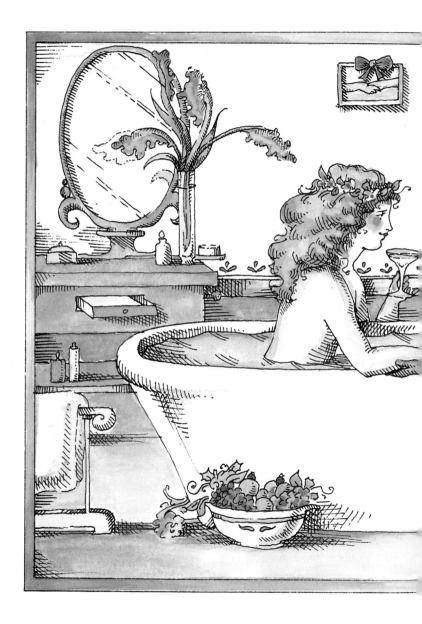

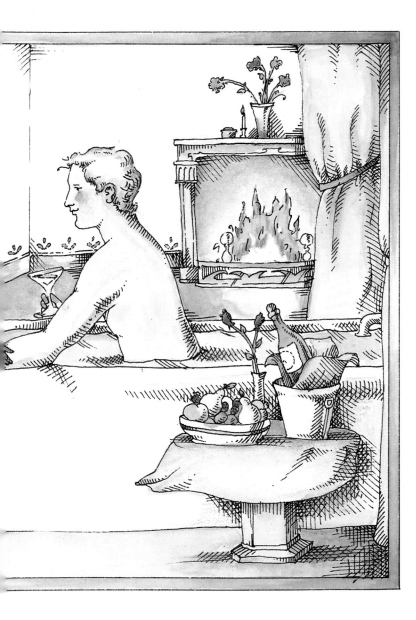

The Valentine Bath

The rose, of course, is the symbol of true love. Here is a recipe for a simple rose water bath . . . embellish it as you desire.

1 oz. essence of rose   1½ qt. distilled water

Mix and add liberally to bath water for a refreshing and romantic bath. Sprinkle rose petals on the surface of the water, and exchange vows of love in this aromatic bath.

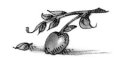

Adam and Eve Bath

This wonderful apple bath will make you feel as if you have stepped back into the Garden of Eden.

¼ cup dried apples   ¼ cup lavender

dried peel of 1 apple   ½ tsp. cinnamon

1½ cups water

Steep ingredients in boiling water for 20 minutes, and add to warm bath water. Keep a bowl of chilled apples by the tub to tempt your lover.

Strawberry Champagne Bath

This is a bath for a special occasion. Make sure you have lots of fresh strawberries on hand to be nibbled throughout the bath.

1 or 2 bottles of your favorite champagne

1 cup fresh strawberry juice

2 or more baskets of fresh strawberries

Add champagne and strained strawberry juice to warm bath water. This fragrant, astringent bath will sooth your skin. It is delicious in more ways than one. Save a glass or two of the champagne to be sipped while soaking.

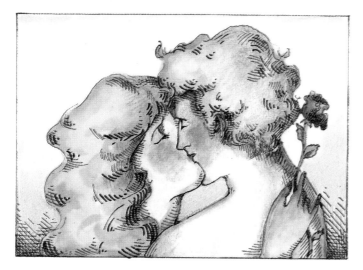

If you have never shared a bath, now is the time to try. Like all great pleasures, it takes thought and careful preparation. For the bath itself, you will need sponges, loofa, gentle brushes, oils and lotions for massage. Bath scents should be carefully selected to appeal to both parties. The room will need attention. Dim the room and fill it with candlelight. If you like, select music which is passionate but not intrusive. You are setting a romantic mood. Try floating whole gardenias, carmelias, or lilies in the water. Keep sparkling wine on hand with bowls of cherries, berries or grapes. Anything simple and sweet will add to the enjoyment of the bath.

If you feel adventuresome, try a theme bath. A Roman bath can be made by using an olive oil massage, white towels and wraps, and white wine following the bath. A French Baroque bath can be made with rose petals, perfume, champagne, and music from the court of Louis XIV. Let your imagination carry you; the possibilities are limitless.

The Persian Bath

Imagine you and your lover are cloistered away in a Persian garden while bathing in this scented water.

1 cup rose petals	*¹/₂ cup rose leaves*
1 tsp. cinnamon	*1 tsp. nutmeg*
¹/₂ tsp. cloves	*2¹/₂ cups water*

Steep ingredients in boiling water for 30 minutes, strain and add to warm bath water. Have scented oil on hand for gentle massage while bathing.

The Anise Bath

This is a heady and romantic fragrance, enjoyed by men and women. Licorice root may be substituted for anise seeds.

¹/₄ cup jasmine tea	*¹/₄ cup anise seeds*	*2 cups water*
¹/₄ cup rose petals	*¹/₄ cup mint leaves*	

Prepare a bath sachet for the ingredients and steep in boiling water for 10 minutes. Add to warm bath water.

Comfort and Joy

This is a wonderful recipe for massage cream, which can bring sensual delight to any shared bath. It is sweet and gentle and very soothing.

2 tsp. lanolin	*1 tsp. honey*
3 oz. witch-hazel	*3 tsp. comfrey water*

Beat ingredients over a double boiler until creamy. Allow to cool. Refrigerate in a glass jar until ready to use. Massage directly onto skin while in the bath.

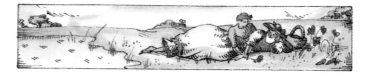

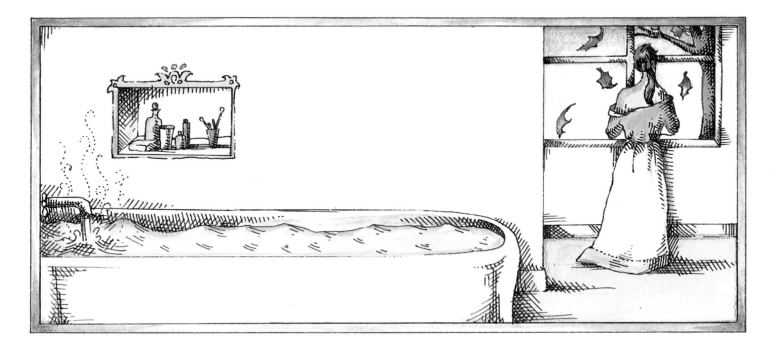

The Fall Bath

n autumn, the light begins to change and the leaves begin to turn. The weather is fickle; one week it's Indian summer, and the next week a sudden frost crisps the air. Leaves turn brilliant hues of red and gold. The air is crisp. We are filled with energy and anticipation of the holidays and the coming cold. Fall is invigorating.

Bathing in Autumn can be wonderfully warming. There is nothing better than a good soak with a good book while the wind howls outside. Remember how good it feels to step out of a steaming tub and snuggle up in flannel?

It is especially important to take good care of your skin in the fall. After a summer in the sun and fresh air, your limbs are back in heavy sweaters and long stockings. The wind and indoor heat will dry out your skin, so be sure to use moisturizers and allow your skin to breathe. Don't be too hasty to don your long johns after a bath. Wrap yourself loosely in a towel and let the air circulate around you. This can be an opportunity to keep skin soothed and in the pink.

The Buttermilk Bath

This will make a wonderfully soothing and moisturizing bath for chilly Fall days.

½ cups buttermilk   *¼ cup orange flower water*

2 tsp. almond oil

Combine ingredients, heat gently, and pour under fast-running bath water.

The Gentleman's Bath

The combined scents in this recipe are particularly pleasing to men, but I like it too.

½ oz. sage   *½ oz. lavender*

½ oz. thyme   *½ oz. savory*

¼ cup salt   *1 garlic bulb (optional)*

1 qt. white vinegar

Steep combined ingredients for 3 weeks. Strain and add ¼ to ½ cup to hot bath water.

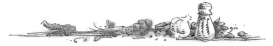

Hot Ginger Friction Rub

This is a great way to warm up quickly after a cold Autumn day. The rub promotes circulation and softens the skin.

3 Tbsp. almond oil   *2 Tbsp. witch-hazel*

1 cup water   *½ oz. fresh or powdered ginger*

Steep ginger in boiling water for 20 minutes. Mix 3 to 4 tablespoons of the ginger water with the oil and witch-hazel and massage directly into wet skin while in the tub. Use a loofah, brush or coarse cloth to massage lotion in briskly. Remaining ginger water may be added to bath if desired.

Fragrant Oatmeal Bath

This is one of the most soothing baths for the skin you can take. Oatmeal has been used for years as a remedy for itching, chafed skin.

3 cups oatmeal   *¼ cup lavender*

¼ cup almond meal

Combine ingredients and grind in a mortar and pestle until it is the consistency of coarse powder. Tie the powder in a bath sachet and suspend under fast-running bath water. The sachet may be added to bath water for a more potent effect.

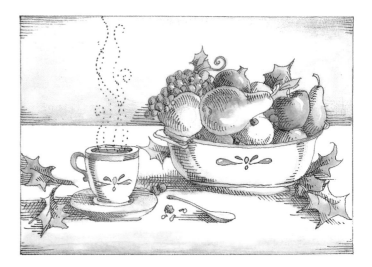

Along with a warming bath, sip a warming cup. Fall is harvest time and the markets are full of fruits which are delicious when made into hot beverages. Pomegranate, apple, pear, grape, and berry juices are delectable when warmed, and you may add a touch of clove or cinnamon or even a shot of brandy. A warm drink in a warm tub will promote a healthy sweat. Be sure to bathe in a heated room, and your fall bath will be complete.

The Foot Bath

f you have never experienced the cheering effect of a foot bath, you are in for a treat. Every waitress or Fuller Brush man knows the joy of coming home to a pan full of warm water for weary feet. Hot or cold, a foot bath will revive your whole body, not just your toes.

These recipes can be used in commercial vibrating foot tubs, or in a plain wash tub. Either way, you'll feel refreshed.

Pine Foot Bath

It is a great way to get started in the morning. It can help promote sleep at night, too.

2 drops pine oil	1 oz. rosemary
1 tsp. almond oil	1 pt. water

Steep ingredients in boiling water for 10 minutes, strain, and add to warm water. This bath is very effective as a cold refresher. Simply add the cooled brew to a pan full of cold water, and stand in it for 2-3 minutes.

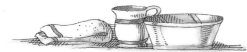

Lavender Foot Bath

This is a stimulating foot bath. After soaking, use a pumice stone to smoothe away calluses — it leaves feet feeling soft.

2 oz. lavender	1 oz. sage
1/2 oz. thyme	1 tsp. sea salt

Place herbs and salt in a large bowl. Add boiling water, and cover. Let set for 1/2 hour, strain, and add to warm water for a brisk foot bath.

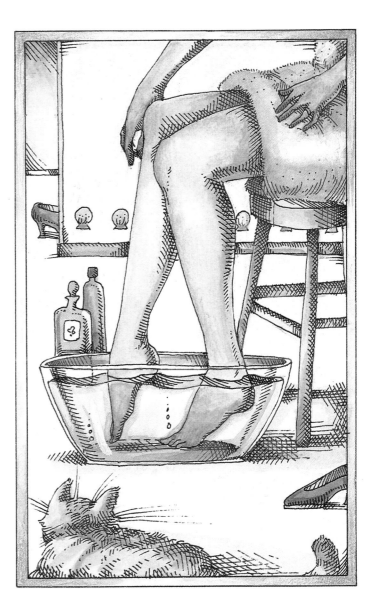

The Twilight Bath

 ne weekday afternoon, as the sun was setting, I celebrated "twilight" in the bath. I lit candles, opened the windows, and settled back to watch the night unfold. As I soaked, there was a knock at the door. It was my neighbor Becky looking for a cup of cream to finish the shortcake she was baking for her kids. "I'm in here Becky." When she found me in the tub, she laughed. "What are you doing taking a bath at this hour?" "I'm celebrating the sunset." I replied. "Well, if I did such a thing, Ed, the kids, the cats and the dog would think I'd jostled my marbles...they expect to find me in the kitchen at this hour." "Exactly the reason you should take off and try one." I said. After thinking for a minute or two Becky decided it was a good idea. Now, once a week, Ed and the kids cook dinner while Becky takes a twilight bath; and now she and I are known to her family as "The Ladies of Leisure."

A bath at sundown can be one of the most relaxing and special of all. After a busy day, you can let go of all your tensions and really enjoy tranquility.

The Blessed Bath

This wonderful sachet will relax you and soothe any blues away. It is also an aid for insomnia.

1 oz. rose petals   *1/2 oz. dried mint*

1 pinch crushed cloves

Tie the ingredients in a bath sachet, and allow to brew under fast-running bath water. Treat yourself to a sip of wine while bathing. Be careful not to overindulge, and your bath will be a happy one.

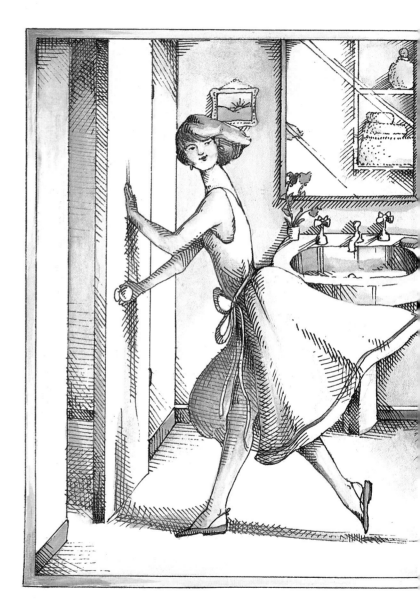

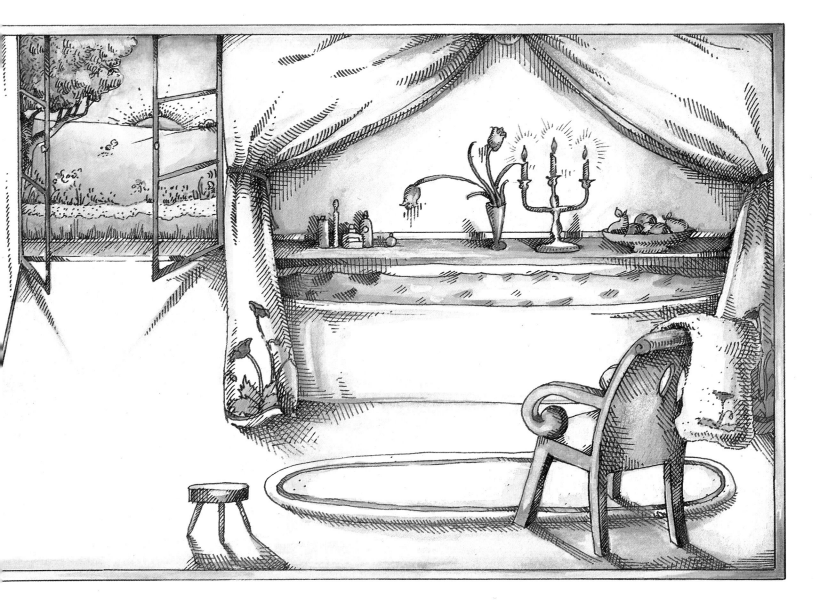

The Bubble Bath

Close your eyes and imagine the most romantic bath in the world...it is probably a bubble bath. Movies have long celebrated stars in bubbles. Cecil B. DeMille was the first director to use the bathtub extensively in movies. Bathtubs were a way to bring the gods and goddesses of the silver screen into the everyday world. In filming his version of *Cleopatra,* he went so far as to have Claudette Colbert steep in an elegant tub filled with asses' milk, just like the real Cleopatra. Other actresses appeared in baths; Gloria Swanson, Greer Garson, Elizabeth Taylor, and Marilyn Monroe to name a few. Great comedians like Charlie Chaplin and Harold Lloyd used bathtubs in their movies, too. Bubble baths for films were made with special bubbling solutions which were effervescent, and produced enough bubbles to hide a multitude of sins.

Everything associated with elegant bathing includes bubbles. Sadly, bubbles can be misused. Bubbling solutions contain chemicals which dry the skin and disturb its acid-mantle. I recommend no more than one bubble bath a week. Balance the rest of the week with an astringent bath and moisturizers, and your skin will stay healthy.

Here are two recipes for bubbling baths. The first includes an herb called soapwort or Fuller's herb. It has been used for centuries as a natural soap. When crushed and mixed with water, it lathers. This lathering agent is called saponin. Homemade herbal bubble baths may not foam as well as store-bought products, but will be much kinder to your skin. The second recipe requires a mild liquid soap solution; gentle dish soap or shampoo will work fine.

Rose and Milk Bubble Bath

Milk is very soothing to the skin and is a natural moisturizer.

> 1½ tsp. grated Soapwort   ¾ cup milk
> ½ cup rose petals

Combine the rose petals and milk, and allow to set overnight in the refrigerator. Before bathing, strain the milk, and add the powdered soapwort. Add to fast-running bath water.

Jasmine Bubble Bath

Jasmine is a classic fragrance. You may substitute the oil of any flower or herb, as you desire.

> 1 Tbsp. mild liquid soap   2 tsp. oil of Jasmine
> 2 tsp. witchhazel

Combine ingredients and add directly to fast-running bath water. This is a particularly fragrant and refreshing bath.

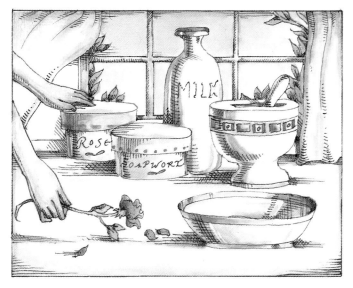

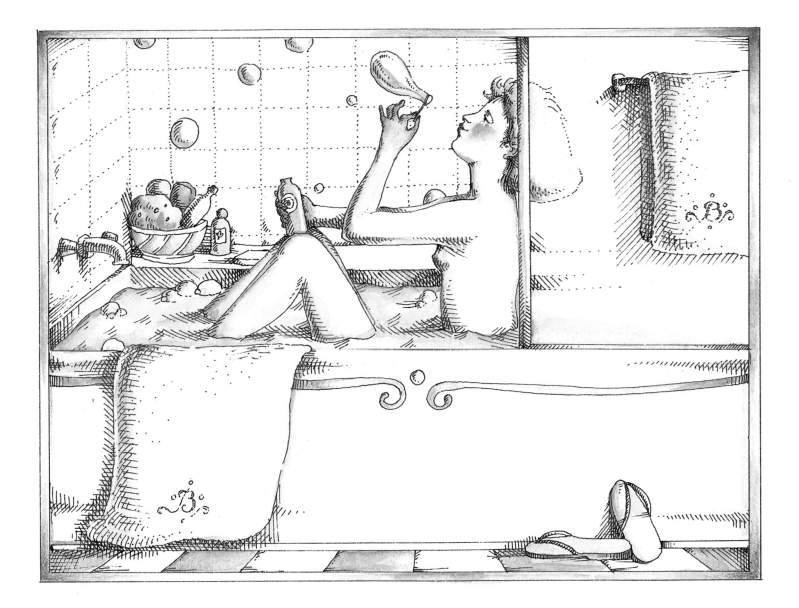

The Extravagant Bath

ntil now we have considered the subtler delights of bathing. Now is the time to try an outrageous bath! Don't be afraid to let your fantasies run away with you.   Great beauties and great lovers have always languished in extravagant and beautiful baths. Marie Antoinette took two baths a day, one to cleanse, the other to rinse and rest in. She had two magnificent tubs made of marble and porcelain. They were fitted with silk curtains, and had gilt fittings and sculpted pedestals. Casanova's tub was portable. It could be transported to his bedside and was big enough for two. Beau Brummel bathed in milk. Mary Queen of Scotts bathed in the wine. Think of these and other celebrated lovers when you are inspired to create an extravagant bath.

Candlelight sets the mood. Sprinkle flower petals around the room and on the surface of the water. Drape the windows with silk. Light incense. Braid pearls in your hair. Fill the room with flowers. Bathe alone, or share the fantasy.

The White Chocolate Bath

For anyone who loves chocolate, this will be the supreme bath experience. It will fill the room with the glorious aroma of chocolate, while cleansing your skin in creamy milk. Add more milk or cream if you desire.

2½ cups milk or cream	1 tsp. oil of chocolate
2 tsp. almond oil	1 pinch cinnamon

Combine ingredients and heat over a double boiler for 5 minutes. Do not boil. Add to fast-running bath water.

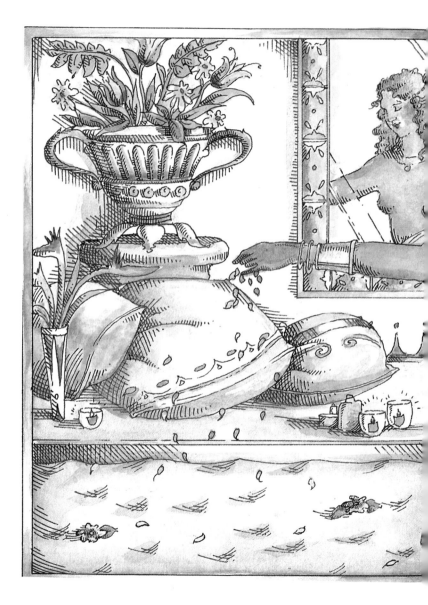

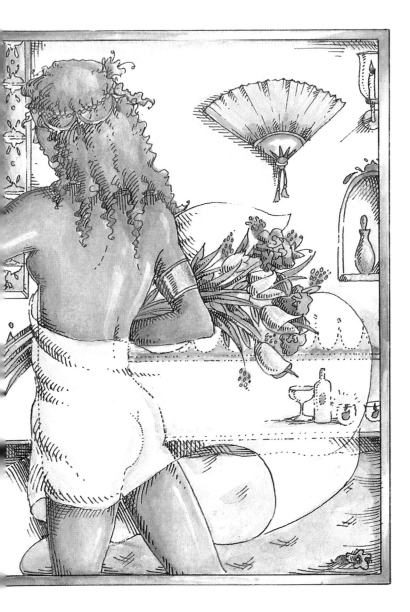

Mary Queen of Scots' Wine Bath

Mary Queen of Scots enjoyed bathing in wine and insisted that it preserved her beauty. It is thought that the wine helped adhere the heavy face powders and rouges which were fashionable at the time. In any case, her habit was so demanding that the Earl of Shewsbury was forced to ask the government to increase her allowance in order to support the habit.

1 or 2 bottles of your favorite wine

Wine is astringent and is safe to bathe in, even in large quantities. If you want a full wine bath, go ahead, but be sure to rinse thoroughly afterwards.

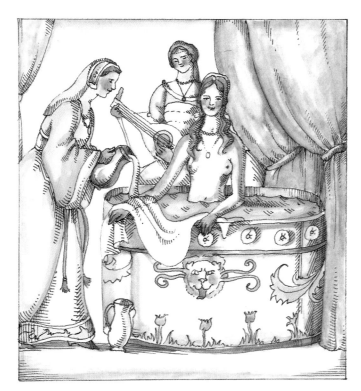

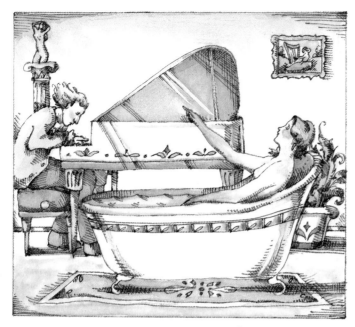

George Sand's Replenishing Milk Bath

The Baroness Aurore Dudevant was a famous novelist and patroness of 19th century France. She was notorious for her affair with Fredrick Chopin, and for being the first woman to smoke and wear trousers in public. She was famous for her wit and intelligence, and her beautiful skin. Her secret for maintaining a lovely complexion was to bathe frequently in milk and honey with a touch of salt. Here is her recipe for an extravagant beauty bath.

3 oz. bicarbonate of soda   *8 oz. salt*

3 lbs. honey   *3 qts. milk*

1 qt. water

Combine salts and soda in the water. Dissolve honey in the milk. Pour salt solution into a tubful of warm bath water, and then slowly stir in the milk and honey.

The Champagne Bath

Sir George Lefevre, author of *Life of a Traveling Physician,* 1843, bathed in champagne in a spa in Brucknau and described it as "A luxury of the first order. It was delicious just to lie still and feel the carbonic escaping all around."

1 or 2 bottles of your favorite champagne

Add the champagne to the bath, but save a glass or two to sip while indulging in the bath. It is safe to bathe in a full champagne bath, like Sir Lefevre, but be sure to rinse thoroughly with clean water afterward.

Berry Baths

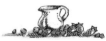

Great beauties throughout history have bathed in the juices of berries. Madame Tallien bathed in crushed strawberries, and afterward sponged perfumed milk over her limbs. Try adding a quart of strawberry juice to warm water. It is naturally astringent. Or . . .

2 cups crushed raspberries   *2 cups fresh cream*

Combine ingredients and sponge over limbs and body while bathing. Add remaining nectar to the water. Rinse thoroughly with clean water following the bath.

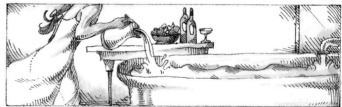

Sparkling Water Bath

NOTE:

For a marvelously refreshing soak, make a bath of your favorite sparkling mineral water. Extravagant though it may be, it will cool and refresh in a mid-summer swelter.

The Dry Bath

 ome of you may feel that less is best: less fuss and less getting wet. If so, try a dry bath, or "sponge bath." I'm sure you remember being bathed this way by your mother when you had a cold as a child.

It is important to sponge bathe in a heated room. You don't want to catch a chill. Fill the sink with hot water, and scent it if you like. Lemon and ginger infusions make marvelous sponge baths. They are both fragrant and stimulating. Use a wash cloth, hand mit, or sponge with soap to start. Wash the upper body first and work your way out from the torso to the arms. Dry yourself immediately and cover up. Then attend to the lower body.

Sponge baths are good for people with arthritis, or temporary disabilities like broken bones or sprains. The stimulating rub can revive aching muscles and will improve circulation.

Try a sponge bath during a hectic day. It takes only minutes and really will give you a lift.

Hot Lemon Sponge Bath

This recipe for a bath sachet makes a heavenly sponge bath, and works well in a tub as well. It is good for people recovering from a cough or cold.

2 Tbsp. fresh grated or powdered ginger	*1 cup water*
2 Tbsp. lemon juice	*1 lemon wedge*

Tie the lemon wedge and ginger in a 3-inch square of muslin, and steep in boiling water for 10 minutes. Fill the sink with hot water. Add the lemon juice and scented infusion. Bathe in a warm room with a washcloth or sponge.

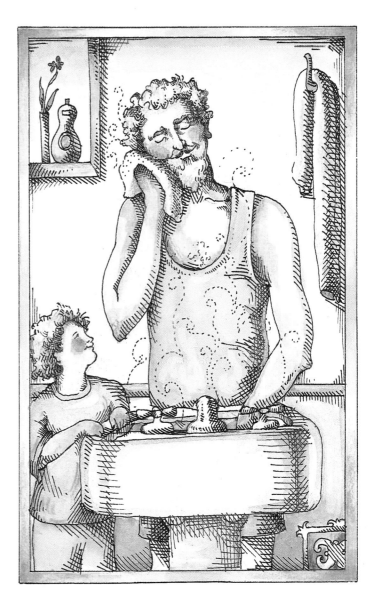

The Winter Bath

id the chill of a wintry day in a steaming tub. It is wonderful to steep indoors while snow falls outside. Central heating and hot water at the tap have made winter bathing a luxury. Imagine life without it. After a day of trudging through icy rain in four layers of clothing, there is no greater pleasure than unpeeling in a toasty room while the tub fills with steam and hot water. It is the warmest place in the house.

Reading in the bath is personal business. I find two things a must; a bath pillow at the head, and plenty of hot water at the tap. Bath trays are available that span the tub and allow you to read without wetting the pages. But I prefer the old fashioned method...wet hands or no. There is nothing more disappointing than settling in with a good book, and feeling your genial tub invaded by lukewarm water. Make sure your water heater has been reset to accommodate the winter months. A hot bath should range from 93–112° F., and is very relaxing. If you wish to soak for longer than 20 minutes, it will be necessary to bathe in cooler water. Hot water baths should be taken when you are unwinding, and should be fairly short.

It is a good idea to stimulate circulation in a winter bath. Some modern bathtubs come with built-in jets or whirlpools, but a simple friction rub will do. Try a salt rub, or use your loofah or brush. Skin can suffer in winter from drying wind and cold. After rising from the tub, pat your skin dry, and apply a moisturizer while skin is still damp. This will help hold moisture in, and will help skin stay soft and healthy.

Spicy Clove Bath

At sunset, steep in this hot-spiced winter bath. Add candlelight to the room, and sip a mug of hot cider.

2 cups rosewater	*½ oz. crushed cloves*
2 bay leaves	*2 cups wine vinegar*

Combine ingredients and boil for 1 hour, adding more water to the original level as it boils down. Store for a week in a cool dark place. Add ½ cup to warm bath water, or combine 1 part vinegar to 8 parts water for a delightful bath splash.

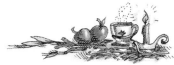

Simple Rosemary Bath

This is one of my favorite baths. Rosemary is a very fragrant and stimulating herb when infused in bath water, and will refresh you after a long, frosty afternoon.

2 oz. rosemary	*2 cups water*

Combine ingredients and boil. Let set for 15 minutes and add to bath water. Add one or two teaspoons of bath oil if your skin is feeling dry.

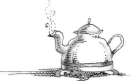

Ginger Tea Bath

This is a wonderfully fragrant bath. It is good to breathe in the steam of this bath to ease tightness in the chest due to asthma or cold weather.

1–2 oz. fresh ginger	*2 tsp. lemon juice*
2 cups water	

Combine and boil ingredients. Let set for 15 minutes and add to warm bath water. A bath sachet may be made of the ginger and added to the bath for a stronger aroma.

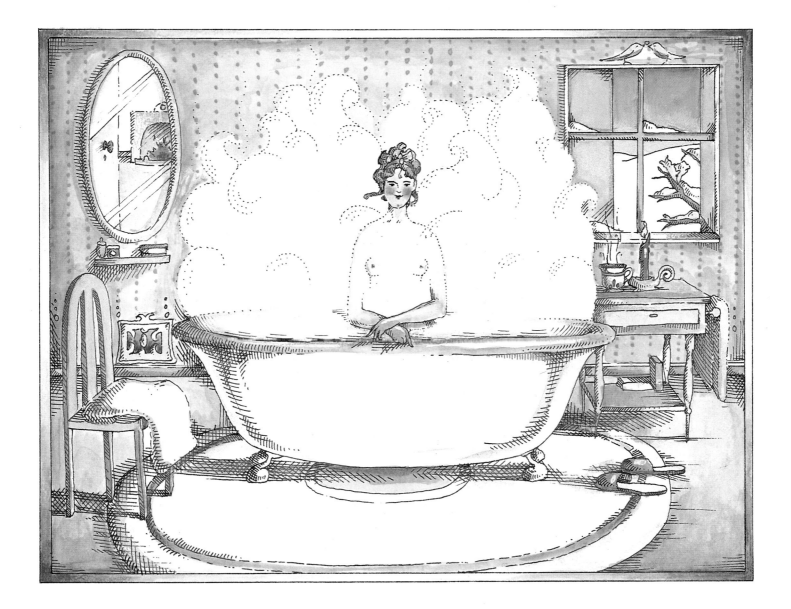

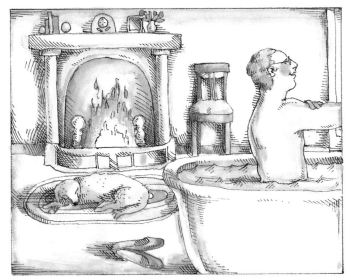

Salt baths have been used in spas for hundreds of years to invigorate and promote circulation. They provide the same wonderful stimulation as a dip in the ocean. And, since you cannot bring the ocean to your tub, do the next best thing: a salt rub. You'll find it a welcome relief from cold or winter nights.

Nautical Salt Bath

Before plunging in, rub a handful of moistened salts on limbs and torso. Be careful to avoid the face, and any areas where skin may be sensitive. Now settle in and soak.

½ cup sea salt, coarse salt, or epsom salt

½ cup water

When rubbing salt on limbs and torso, wet salt but do not saturate. For an alternative to the rub, add a few teaspoons of salt to warm bath water. Be sure to moisturize thoroughly after a salt bath. And remember to rinse the tub thoroughly when you're through.

Tokyo Salt Bath

Seaweed is refreshing when added to bath water. It is soothing to skin.

2 tsp. sea salt, coarse salt, or epsom salt

1 oz. dried seaweed   1 oz. dried kelp

Make a bath sachet of the kelp and seaweed, and let it suspend under fast-running bath water. Add the salt and sachet to the water for a refreshing and warming bath. Use a brush or loofa to stimulate circulation.

Hollywood Salt Bath

Imagine yourself soaking in the sun under the swaying palms of Hollywood as you enjoy this aromatic citrus salt bath.

½ cup sea salt, coarse salt or epsom salt

peel of 1 lemon   2 drops oil of lemon or orange

Combine ingredients, and let set overnight. Add a handful of the scented salt to warm bath water.

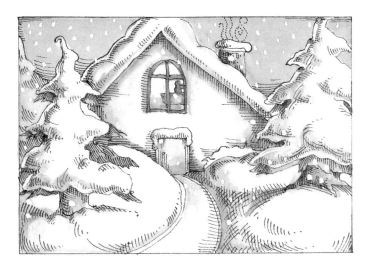

Outdoor Bathing

Bathing outdoors in the dead of winter may seem crazy but it has been practiced with enthusiasm for centuries, In Russia, the first baths were ceremonial, and took place in frozen lakes and rivers. The Tsar was sprinkled each new year with water from the Neva River. Newborn babies were dunked in the freezing water, and those who survived were blessed for a long life. Today, the Russians are fond of hot steam baths followed by a plunge in a cold pool or river, or even the snow. The Finns beat themselves with birch branches in a hot room to promote circulation before taking a roll in the snow.

If you want to try a winter bath outdoors, be sure to consult your doctor first. Bathing in cold water can be bracing, and may jolt your system. If you are in good health, and enjoy something different, give it a try. Just be sure to bathe wisely.

Hot tubs in winter are a real treat. Don't soak too long and wrap yourself well after rising from the tub. Sudden changes of temperature are stimulating for your body, and must be experienced with care and common sense.

For a special treat — bathe in hot water with a glass of chilled vodka or Perrier. The combination of hot water, chilly air, and cold drink will give your body a lift.

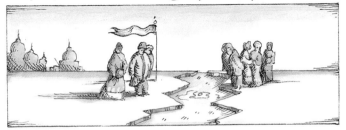

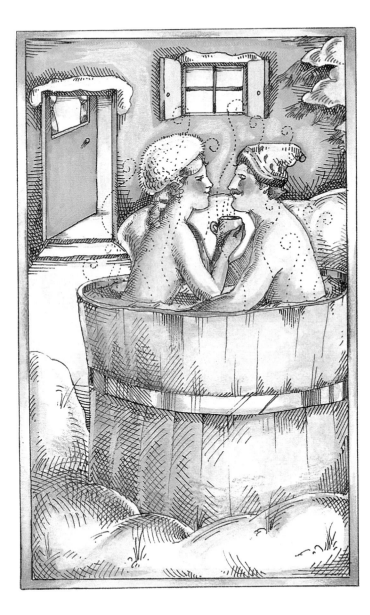

The Moon Bath

 wynne and Peter moved from a quiet country house to the city last year. I was sorry to see them go. It was a career move for them, and I knew it would make them happy. One month after the move Gwynne began to call very late at night. She couldn't sleep. "It's so different here," she said. "I can't stop worrying about my new job." After a week of our late night talks, I had an idea. "When you hang up, I want you to draw a warm bath, and settle in until you feel drowsy. Let your thoughts go. Just relax."

I discovered the benefits of midnight bathing in college, when the kids in my dormitory romped every night until two in the morning. A midnight bath was just the thing for frazzled nerves.

I didn't hear from Gwynne for a month, and then I received a mysterious package. It contained a beautiful porcelain jar filled with rose petals, and a letter. Here is what it said. "Dear Cathy, your suggestion of a midnight bath has rescued me from my misery. That night, I filled the tub and settled in. Soon, Peter wandered in to see what I was up to. Before we knew it, we were taking a midnight bath together every night. Sometimes we light candles, and listen to music. It's heavenly. We're sleeping again and everything is looking up. Please come stay with us soon . . . and thanks for being there. Love, Gwynne."

You need not wait until sleeping is a problem to enjoy a midnight bath. Surprise someone you love with a sensual midnight massage. It is an opportunity to try exotic oils and new fragrances. They can be soothing, romantic, and a blessing for nerves any time.

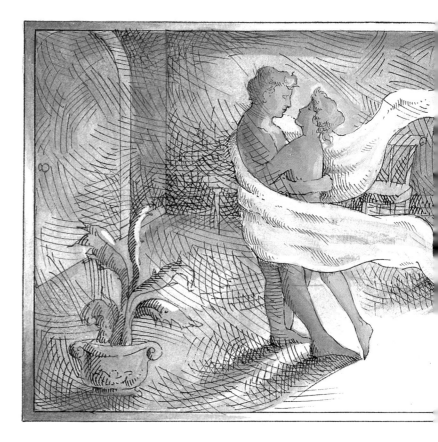

Jasmine Bath

Jasmine flowers have one of the most beautiful and romantic fragrances in the world. This makes a very romantic and soothing midnight bath. Think of bathing in a pool near a vine of night-blooming jasmine.

2 drops oil of Jasmine   *1 cup distilled water*

Combine ingredients and add to warm bath water. Float whole camellias or gardenias on the surface of the water.

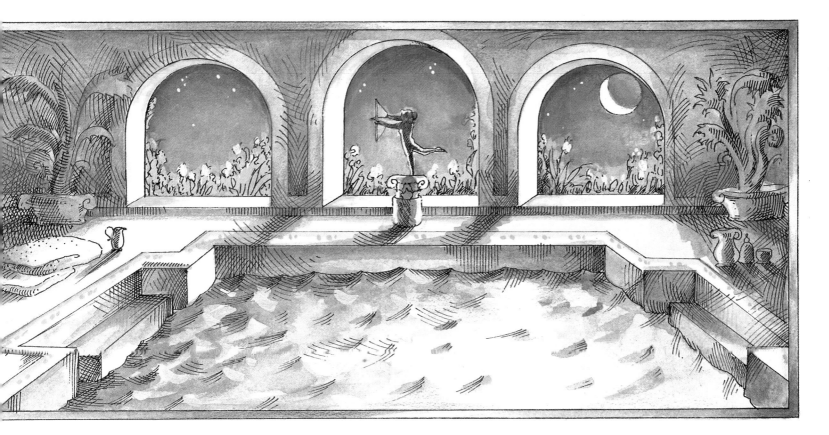

Magnolia Bath

Magnolia is a flower with a potent and evocative scent. It is particularly effective at night.

1 cup magnolia flowers   ½ cup alcohol

½ cup distilled water

Steep combined ingredients in sunlight for a week or two, or until liquid has taken on the scent of the flower. Add to warm bath water as desired.

Fresh Spruce Bath

This bath will fill the room with the scent of a pine forest in cool moonlight. It is a wonderful fragrance.

2–3 lbs. young spruce twigs or green cones   4 gal. water

Combine ingredients and let set 12-24 hours. Then boil for 2 hours. Add liberally to warm bath water. May be used as an air freshener as well.

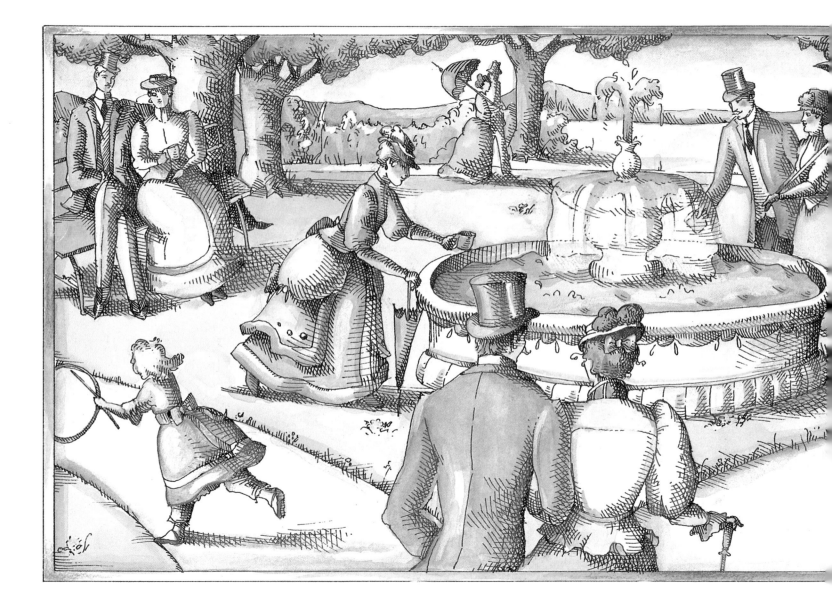

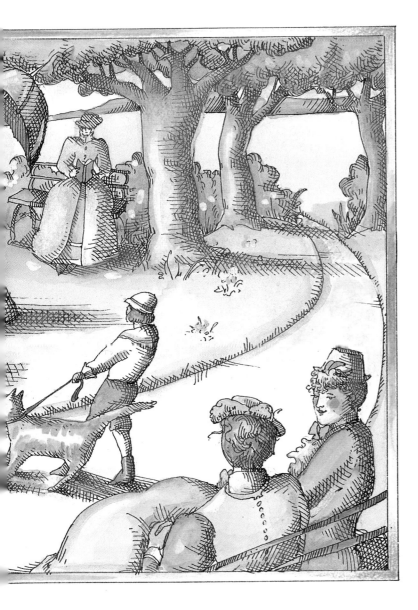

Curative Baths

rom ancient times to the present, people have looked to water for cures. The first bath resorts were founded on natural springs, and were elaborate temples dedicated to the gods of water. People flocked to them for every conceivable cure.

The tradition of going to water for treatment was perfected in Europe. Spas were used to treat everything from broken bones and nervous exhaustion to diseases of the heart, lungs, brain, and blood. Many of these centers, like Lourdes, were the sites of miracles; others for the mysterious curative powers of the water alone. Water was taken both internally and was bathed in.

The word "spa" comes from the resort of Spa at Ardennes, founded in 1326. But the word did not come into use until 1342, when Emperor Charles IV discovered the great Bohemian spa at Carlsbad. By 1351 there were so many visitors there, it was necessary to impose a "cure tax." Beethoven and Goethe convalesced there. Carlsbad claimed to have cured more illnesses than any other spa in Europe, even occult disorders.

Bath in England is one of Europe's most famous spas. Its origin is Roman, but the waters have been enjoyed throughout history. Bathers there had the exclusive pleasure of having prayers written for them by the Bishop of Bath. In 1449, the Bishop stated that anyone who had reached puberty was required to wear drawers and a robe while bathing. Another Bishop preached that "God must heal the Waters before they have any virtue to heal you." Queen Anne of Denmark visited Bath three times, and claimed it cured her of all her ills.

Baden in Switzerland had an entirely different atmosphere. There, men, women and children bathed together. The sexes were separated only by a thin partition (sometimes with little holes in it); and entered the baths in full view of one another. It was a spa with high spirits.

By the 18th century, spas were places where the elite came to be seen and to "take the waters." Napoleon went to Vichy, George Frederick Handel went to Aix-la-Chapelle, Queen Victoria preferred Aix-les-Bains, and Robert Burns was sent to the sea at Solway. Each spa had its own reputation. During the day one took the cure, the evening was a time for dining, dancing and gambling.

In 1808 the spa at Baden-Baden established a gambling bank to attract wealthy patrons from Europe and abroad. By 1830 Baden-Baden had approximately 15,000 visitors a year. The spa had a reputation for "morality . . . of a very low standard . . .," where ladies were seen at the gambling tables and gentlemen flaunted their mistresses in public. Casinos are still very much a part of the social life of modern spas.

Although life was elegant and refined after dark, taking the cure was often an ordeal.

Water was sipped by the gallon, and due to the high mineral content, it often smelled horrible! People were encouraged to drink water throughout the day to cure everything from gall stones to sprains. The most strenuous cures were external ones. Arm baths, Dripping Sheet Baths, Dry Blanket Packs, Douche Baths, Electric Baths, Foot Packs, Head Baths, Gargling Baths, Hot Air Baths, Mud Baths, Nose Baths, Plunge Baths, Rain Baths, Sitz Baths, Vapor Baths, Wet Sheet Baths, Wet Compresses, Slime Baths, Sulfur Baths, Deluge Baths, Spray Baths, and Sweat Baths were offered to the ailing patient. Charles Dickens took his wife to Malvern in England for a cold

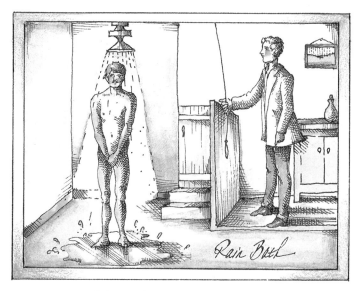

water cure and found ". . . a good deal in it . . . My experience of that treatment induces me to hold that it is wondrously efficacious where there is constitutional vitality; where there is not, I think it may be a little questionable."

To say the least, spa cures were varied and enervating. People who went were seeking balm for body and soul. Most came away satisfied. Whether spas succeeded in curing people did not seem to matter a great deal. It was the experience of getting away from the drudge of day-to-day routine, and if the water helped — more the better.

Spas have continued to operate since before Roman times, while private baths and bathing practices have suffered ups and downs through history. In America and Europe, spas enjoy a thriving business, and provide just about the same variety of conveniences as ancient spas. Although the luxury of taking the waters was once affordable only to the very rich, today's spas are within the reach of anyone who wishes to cleanse, cure and rejuvenate.

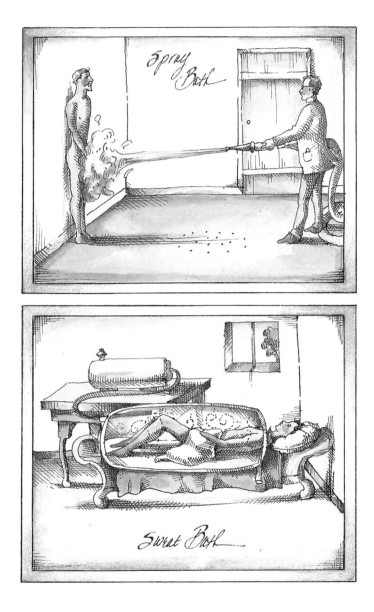

Spray Bath

Sweat Bath

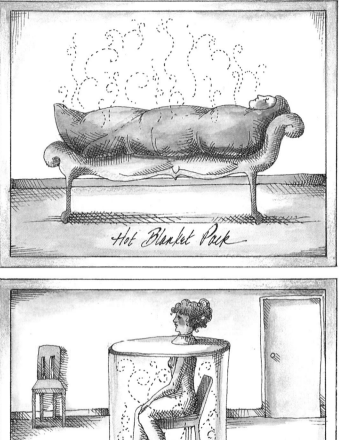

Hot Blanket Pack

Portable Vapor Bath

The Children's Bath

Almost all kids adore bathtime. I've seen tearful babies break into smiles as they are lowered into a warm tub. Some children look forward to bathtime as playtime. There are amazing bath toys available for children of all ages: Ducks, boats, diving frogs, rubber monsters, waterproof books, bath dollhouses, and floating safety chairs.

Bathing infants requires care and common sense. A full bath twice a week is fine in cool weather, as long as the face and diaper area are kept clean. There are special tubs and basinettes designed to cradle an infant securely, but a washbowl, dishpan, or kitchen sink will do. Have a mild soap, wash cloth, towel, powder, and baby oil ready. Water should be shallow and warm (90°). Support the baby with one hand and wash with the other. If the baby is afraid of the water, or you are afraid he will slip, sponge him in your lap. Most babies get over the fear of water in 2 or 3 weeks. Try later with shallow water in a dishpan. Your enthusiasm for the bath will encourage the baby.

Children like to share baths with brothers and sisters, which is fine if the parent keeps a watchful eye. Too much play can lead to slipping and a wet bathroom floor! If your child needs an inducement to take a bath, try bringing toys and games to the tub. Or try carving soap together before the bath. Use a dull butter knife and bars of colored soap to carve animals, people, cars, houses, dinosaurs, or space ships. Bring them to the tub and invent stories. By the age of six, most children want privacy. Parents can use this time to teach children to care for their own bodies and to develop a healthy respect for the privacy of others.

Mild Lettuce Bath

My friend Maria, who has 4 children, recommends this bath for bedtime. It is soothing and promotes sleep.

7 to 10 large Romaine lettuce leaves   *1 qt. water*

Add leaves to boiling water and set for 5 mintues. Strain, and add to warm bath water.

Cucumber Bath

This is a very refreshing and mild bath for children. It can be used any time for any age.

1 cucumber   *¾ cup water*

Slice and peel the cucumber, and place in a bowl. Pour boiling water over the slices and allow to steep until cucumber becomes mushy. Strain, and add the juice to warm bath water.

Baby Powder

Some doctors discourage the use of powders which contain talc. Here is a recipe for unscented baby powder which does not contain talc.

½ cup cornstarch   *½ cup rice flour*

Combine and use liberally after bath and after diapering. May be used by adults as well.

Baby Oil

NOTE:

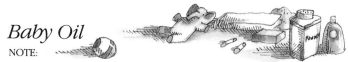

Most store-bought oils are simply mineral oil and fragrance. Plain mineral oil will do just as well and will be less expensive.

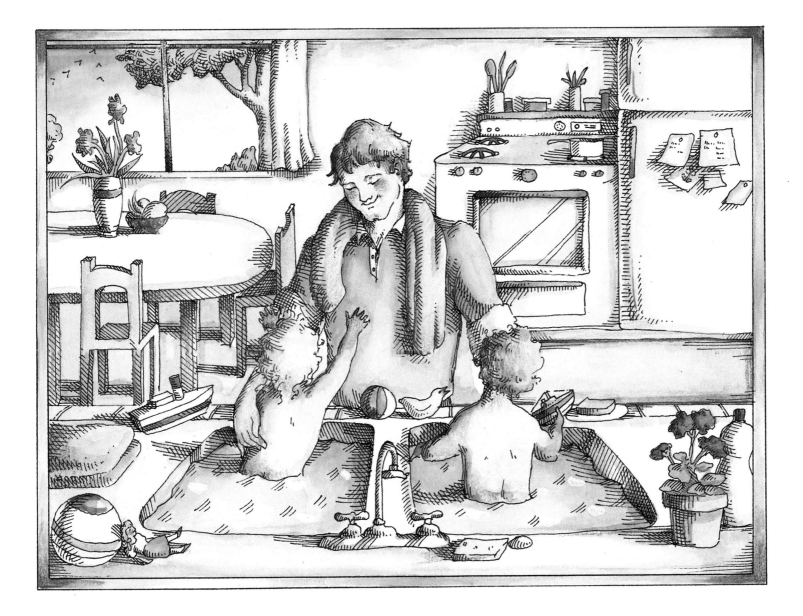

water splash, and make the rubdown a vigorous one. This will stimulate your circulation and send you into the world full of energy. Otherwise, take time to rest while your body adjusts to the air temperature. Pat yourself dry and then wrap yourself loosely in the towel or a cotton robe. Allow the remaining moisture to evaporate slowly.

When you are dry, wrap up in an elegant robe. Men and women can find beautiful cotton, silk, and satin robes in all colors and styles. Many stores have departments which specialize in bath and bedroom fashions. It is an easy way to look and feel superb.

After the Bath

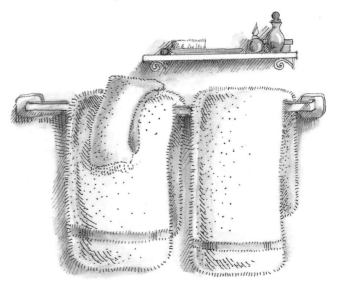

his is one of my favorite times (second only to the bath itself). Halfway between the wet world and the dry, it is a dreamy time. One to languish in. I try to take an hour or so to complete the bath; wrapping up in an Egyptian cotton robe with a good book, or listening to music. It is a luxury well worth the effort.

First you must dry off in a healthy and proper manner. Each member of the family should have a fresh set of towels for every bath. One hand towel and a full bath towel will do. I think cotton terry-cloth towels are best. They are luxurious, thick and absorbent. My favorite after-bath pleasure is to dry off in a warmed towel. There are racks available which gently heat the towel while you bathe.

After you step out of the tub, give yourself a brisk rub-down. If you are in a hurry, finish your bath with a cold

It is a good idea to keep a box or jar of baking soda by the tub along with a special sponge for cleaning. A quick sprinkle of soda and a whisk of the sponge should do the trick. For difficult problems, add a splash of vinegar. These products make fine cleansers and will not spoil the next bath if any residue is left.

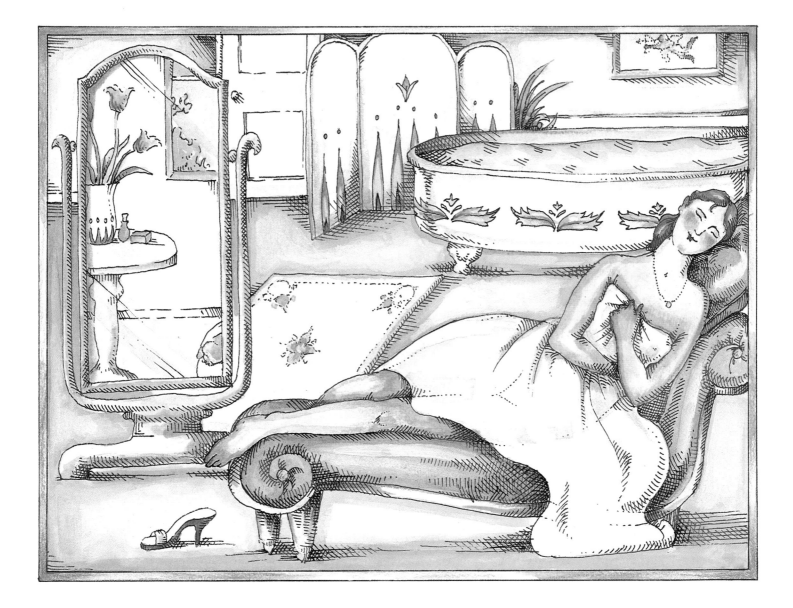

Cold Cream

Cold cream is one of the oldest beauty creams, and was first used by the Greek physician Galen. It received its name from the cool feeling it left upon skin after being applied. It makes a wonderful overnight cream and is superb for removing make-up.

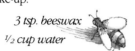

¼ cup mineral oil	*3 tsp. beeswax*
¼ rose petals	*½ cup water*

Steep rose petals in boiling water for 30 minutes. Melt mineral oil and beeswax over a double boiler. Strain the rose water and add ¼ cup to the melted wax and oil, stirring constantly. Pour mixture into a glass jar and refrigerate. After cream has set you may add a drop of food coloring and whip until the cream is smoothe and light. One or two drops of rose oil may be substituted for the rose water.

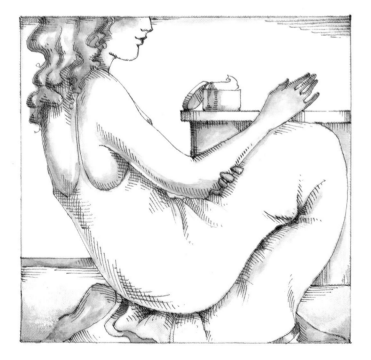

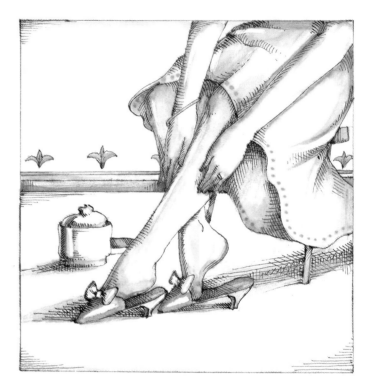

Vanilla Cream Moisturizer

This cream has a similar consistency to cold cream, and is very good for smoothing on elbows, heels, and other problem dry areas. It has a delightful aroma.

½ cup petroleum jelly	*2 tsp. beeswax*
3 tsp. lanolin	*¼ cup water*
½ tsp. vanilla extract	

Melt petroleum jelly and beeswax over a double boiler, and add the lanolin. Carefully stir in the water in a steady stream. Remove the mixture from the double boiler and stir until it has cooled. Add the vanilla extract and refrigerate. When set, whip until creamy.

Moisturizers

eep skin soft and supple by moisturizing after every bath. Oils and creams protect skin by holding water in and by guarding it from drying sun, wind, and cold. It is best to smooth on lotion while your skin is still damp. Pat skin dry. Then apply your moisturizer with gentle massaging strokes to feet, legs, arms, and torso, finishing with upward strokes on the neck and face.

Your face needs special care. Areas around the eyes and cheeks tend to be dry, while the nose, chin, and forehead are not. Use only as much oil or cream as you need to feel comfortable. Too much can cause skin to produce less of its own oil and may result in drier skin. Each person has a different skin type. Delicate, dry or oily: everyone needs a moisturizer to maintain a healthy and youthful complexion.

Store-bought creams are made with mineral oil, water, emulsifiers, and fragrance. Emulsifiers are chemicals which keep the other ingredients mixed. The recipes you find here are simple and fresh, and will work as well as any store-bought product, without the additives or expense.

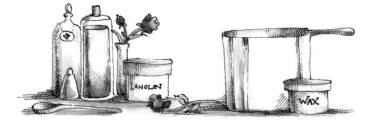

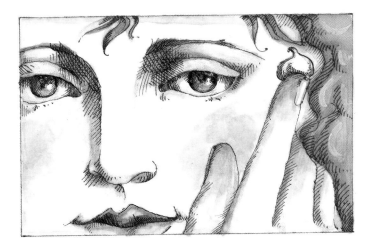

Cucumber Cold Cream

Cucumber juice is a delicate and soothing element when added to a moisturizer. It has been used for centuries for its cooling feel and pleasant scent.

½ cup lanolin	*2 tsp. almond oil*
1 cucumber	*¾ cup water*

Pour boiling water over sliced and peeled cucumber. Let it stand until the cucumber becomes mushy. Strain and keep the juice. Melt lanolin over a double boiler and add the almond oil. Pour in juice in a steady stream. Remove from the double boiler and stir until cool. Refrigerate until needed.

Simple Moisturizer

If you are in a hurry, apply mineral oil directly to the skin, follow these simple instructions.

lanolin	*mineral oil*

Mix equal parts of the oils in a cup until creamy, and apply to moist skin. Lanolin is very gentle and protects well in cold weather.

Colognes

y mother was born in Cologne, Germany, and remembers a fountain in the middle of the city which sprayed eau de cologne for all to dip their hankies in. Eau de cologne was invented by an Italian barber who settled there in the 17th century. This light, refreshing perfume was originally made of the oil of lemons and oranges mixed with the essence of lavender and orange blossom. Today, colognes are made of many different fragrances. Cologne has a high alcohol content, and, when splashed on, leaves the skin feeling cool and revived. Both men and women enjoy this enticing aromatic. It can be worn on casual occasions instead of perfume. The charm of cologne is that it has a refreshing, clean scent which lasts long enough to entice without overpowering.

Colognes are easy to make, are romantic and invigorating, and should be applied with abandon after a bath!

Lemon–Lavender Cologne

This is a scent that evokes the sweet smell of springtime. It can be enjoyed by men and women alike.

³⁄₄ cup alcohol	¹⁄₄ tsp. oil of lemon
1 tsp. oil of lavender	2 drops clove oil or 2 cloves
	¹⁄₄ cup distilled water

Dissolve the oils in alcohol, and add cloves if desired. Then add water. The cologne may be used right away, or may be left to set for a week for a more potent aroma.

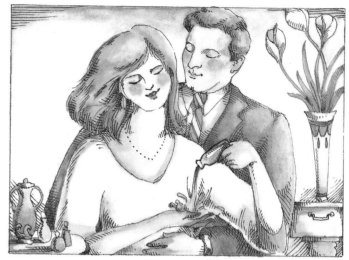

My Summer Cologne

This classic fragrance is based upon a recipe for Hungary water, which is much loved in Europe.

1¹⁄₂ cups alcohol	1¹⁄₄ tsp. rosemary oil
1¹⁄₄ tsp. lemon oil	3 Tbsp. rose essence

Combine oil and alcohol and use directly. Fragrance may be stored in a dark place for 1 week for a more potent scent.

Sandlewood Cologne

This is a heady fragrance especially enjoyed by men.

1¹⁄₂ cup alcohol	¹⁄₄ tsp. oil of sandlewood
2 drops oil of lemon	2 tsp. orange flower water

Combine oils with alcohol, and then add the water. Use directly, or let set for a week for a more potent aroma.

Splashes

 ath splashes are delicate fragrances, which can be poured liberally into bath water or drenched over limbs after the bath. Small amounts of juice from fruits or berries, or essences of flowers are mixed with water to create a splash. Scented vinegars may be used as well. Splashes are very gentle to the skin and are particularly good for people with sensitive or dry skin. Splashes may be used for cleansing, too.

Make enough to use freely after every bath. Try making a different scented splash for every day of the week. Or coordinate the fragrance with the scent used in the bath. Indulge.

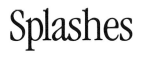

Aloe Splash

Aloe is mild and soothing and can be mixed into water or applied directly to the skin. It makes a delightful splash.

¹/₂ tsp. aloe juice   1 cup water

Combine and use as an after-bath splash, rinse, or cleanser. Recipe may be doubled or tripled as you desire.

Lemon Splash

Lemon is a natural astringent, and makes a fine cleanser.

³/₄ cup witchhazel   3 Tbsp. lemon juice

¹/₂ cup water

Mix and splash liberally in bath water, or after bath.

Blueberry Splash

This is a scented vinegar splash, and may be made with raspberries if you prefer.

¹/₂ cup blueberries   2 cups vinegar

2 tsp. honey   1 piece cinnamon bark

Combine and let stand 2 weeks, shaking the jar daily. Mix 1 part vinegar with 8 parts water as desired for bath splash and cleanser. This scented vinegar may be added to bath water or may be used for cooking.

Cucumber Splash

The juice of the cucumber, when mixed with water, is an excellent cooler and rinse.

1 cup cucumber juice   2 cups water

Slice and peel the cucumber and place it in a bowl. Pour 1 cup boiling water over the slices and allow to steep until cucumber becomes mushy. Strain and mix with the remaining cup of water. This recipe is best when fresh. Refrigerate if you wish to use it later.

NOTE:
Floral splashes may be made by mixing 1 ounce essence of the desired flower with 1 gallon of distilled water. You may mix the floral water into other splashes for a delicately different effect.

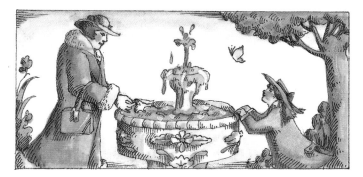

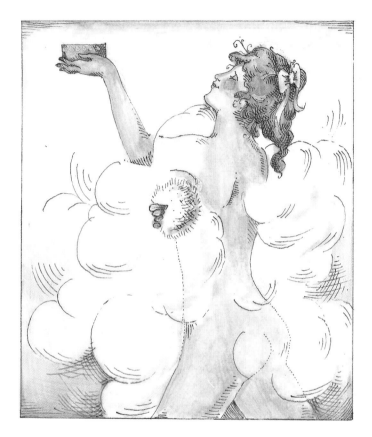

Powders

fter you have towelled yourself dry, moisturized, and applied your favorite splash or cologne, try a light dusting with a delicate bath powder. Scented or unscented powders are one of the great after-bath pleasures. In hot weather, powder will leave skin silky smooth and will help it stay dry and refreshed. In winter, it soothes chafing. Bath powders may be sprinkled from a jar, shaker, or applied with a dusting puff. Men as well as women enjoy an after-bath dust. It is a simple, luxurious finale to a good bath.

Simple Bath Powder

For those of you who prefer an unscented sprinkle, this is the answer. Cornstarch is very absorbant, and rice flour is light and silky. This makes a fine baby powder as well.

¹/₄ cup cornstarch   *¹/₂ cup rice flour*

Combine and sprinkle directly to freshly cleaned skin.

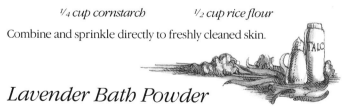

Lavender Bath Powder

Lavender is a classic scent for products used in the tub and after bath.

¹/₄ cup cornstarch   *¹/₄ rice flour*

¹/₄ cup talc   *4 drops oil of lavender*

Drop the oil into the powders and stir. Powder will absorb the scent without becoming sticky. Keep in a moisture-proof container.

Vanilla Bath Powder

Vanilla is one of the richest fragrances for after-bath powder.

¹/₄ cup talc   *¹/₄ cup rice flour*

3 drops vanilla extract or 1 vanilla bean

Combine the flours and add the extract. Stir and place in a moisture-proof container. If vanilla bean is used, place the bean in the container with the powder.

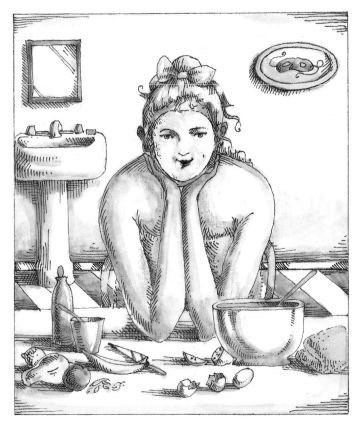

Masks

nce or twice a month, it is a good idea to give yourself a facial treatment beginning with a deep-cleansing mask. Masks may be used by people with dry or oily skin as long as the mask is selected carefully to be compatible with skin type. Pores should be open to promote deep cleansing, so begin by pressing a steaming washcloth to your face. Massage the mask gently over the skin with upward strokes. Then sit back and relax. After 5 or 10 minutes, rinse the mask away with cool water and apply an astringent lotion for a final cleansing. Finish with a moisturizer and you are on your way to enjoying a clear and healthy complexion.

Papaya Facial Scrub

Papaya is filled with enzymes which help cleanse and beautify skin. This mask is recommended for normal or oily skin.

1/2 papaya	*1 egg*
1/2 tsp. lemon juice	

Blend ingredients and apply to the face for 10 minutes.

Banana Face Mask

This slightly abrasive mask is good for removing dry, flaky skin cells. It is a moisturizing mask and is especially good for dry skin.

1 ripe banana	*1 tsp. almond meal*
2 tsp. yogurt	

Mix and massage with upward strokes over face and neck. Leave for 5 to 10 minutes, and rinse thoroughly with cool water.

Oatmeal Facial Scrub

This is a very soothing mask, and is slightly abrasive. It may be used by people with dry or oily skin.

4 tsp. oatmeal	*1 tsp. dried mint*
2 tsp. mineral oil	

Grind oatmeal and leaves into a fine powder, and add oil and enough warm water to make a paste. Apply and let set for 10 minutes. Rinse thoroughly with cool water.

The Facial Steam Bath

y first experience with the benefits of a facial steam bath came at sixteen when I was studying ballet in New York. Nina, a tall blonde dancer with the milkiest complexion I'd ever seen, shared the bus with me each morning. One day I asked her how she kept her skin so beautiful. The havoc caused by humidity, perspiration, and the terrible city air seemed impossible to overcome. She described her regimen this way. Two or three times a month, she ended her day with a facial steam bath. Besides opening pores, it helped eliminate oils and impurities from the skin. She also maintained a careful cleansing and moisturizing routine. And, she drank eight glasses of water a day!

I couldn't keep up with all that water, but I did begin to use a facial steam bath. The results were visible immediately. It proved to be a soothing, enjoyable treatment. A steam bath keeps skin clean and moisturized without damaging elasticity or surface layers. Begin the steam with a clean face, and finish with a moisturizer. Your face will look and feel marvelous.

The Pine Facial Steam

This facial also makes a wonderful humidifier to be inhaled when conjested. It can be used as a room freshener as well.

1 tsp. oil of pine   *1 tsp. mint leaves*   *2–3 cups water*

1 tsp. peppermint   *1 tsp. camomile*

Add the ingredients to a porcelain bowl, pour in boiling water, and continue to steam as long as you desire.

The Lavender Facial Steam

This is a gentle, fragrant steam bath, which will leave you feeling refreshed and relaxed.

¼ cup dried lavender   *peel of 1 lemon, dried*

2 tsp. rosemary

Add the ingredients to the porcelain bowl, pour in boiling water and steam for as long as you wish.

The Floral Facial Steam

Imagine yourself in an Indian garden while taking in the glorious fragrances of this steam.

Combine a pinch of: lavender   *rose petals*

rose buds   *jasmine tea*   *2–3 cups water*

orange peel

Add the ingredients to a porcelain bowl, pour in boiling water, and steam for as long as you wish.

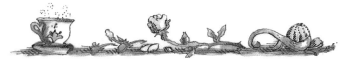

NOTE:

1. You'll need a tea pot, dried herbs and flowers, a bowl, a measuring cup and a towel.

2. Add selected ingredients to the bowl.

3. Boil water.

4. Pour approximately 2 cups of the boiling water into the bowl. Cover and let steep for 5 minutes.

5. Use the towel to tent your head over the bowl; then steam for 5 to 10 minutes.

6. Splash your face with cold water and gently pat dry.

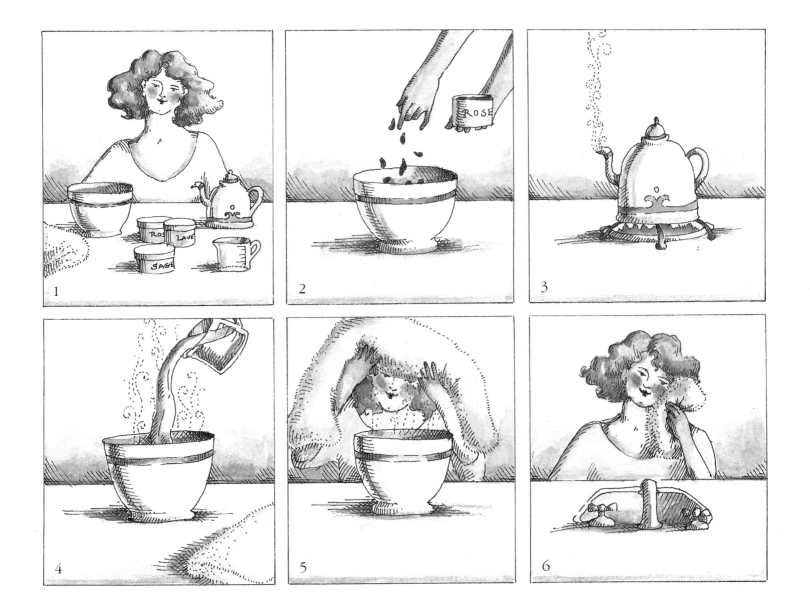

t no other time in history have there been more opportunities for pleasure in the bath. Bath lovers can indulge themselves at home in luxurious private baths or attend spas where the pleasures of bathing are enhanced by Jacuzzis, saunas and massages. Simple or elaborate, short or long, indoors or out, baths have never been so accessible, pleasing, or varied.

Never feel guilty about relaxing in a warm tub. Although cleanliness is a result, it is not the only benefit of bathing. Delicate scents and warm water can soothe your soul as well as your body. Pampering yourself in a beautiful bath is one of life's pleasures! When you are relaxed and re-freshed, work, play and romance flow more easily. If it means you'll indulge yourself more than once a day...do so! Do what pleases you at the moment.

You are now a bath connoisseur. I hope this book and its recipes will inspire you to seek out even greater adven-tures and delights in bathing. It has been my plea-sure...now it can be yours. You know the basic recipes. Embellish your favorites. Invent your own recipes, fra-grances, and bath experiences. Let your imagination go as you soak in a scented tub!

Share the pleasures you have discovered in the bath. These recipes make wonderful gifts. Create your own concoctions, then bottle them with hand-lettered labels and your personal touch. You will be giving someone you care for a special treat. The bath fragrances you invent will be a tempting invitation for a friend to indulge in the luxury of private time spent in the tub.

Take time when the mood strikes to enjoy a bath. Re-member, you are taking care of the most precious gift you possess...your healthy body.

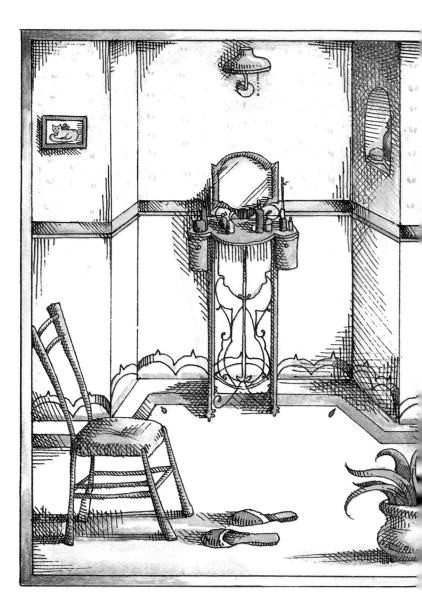

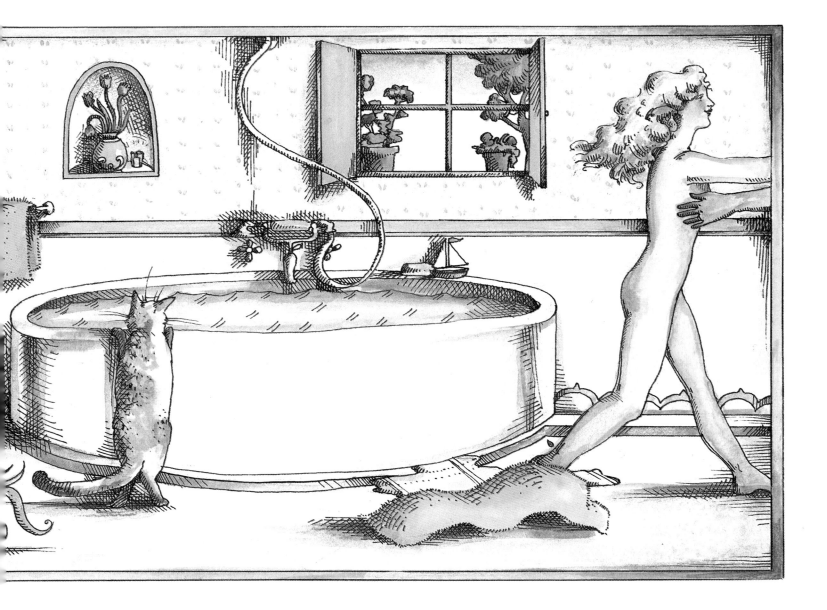

Recipe Index

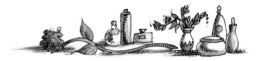

Sources

Ingredients for the recipes in this book can be found in most local health food or gourmet food shops. But if you have trouble finding exactly what you want, or if you wish to buy in bulk, try ordering from one of the following mail-order sources. They will be happy to send you a catalogue (sometimes for a nominal fee). You may select plants, seeds, dried ingredients, and essential oils. No matter where you live, there is a distributor within reach.

Aphrodisia Products Incorporated (dried ingredients & essential oils)
45 Washington Street
Brooklyn, New York 11201 (718) 852–1278

Caswell-Massey Co. Ltd. (dried ingredients & essential oils)
Catalogue Division
111 Eighth Avenue
New York, New York 10011 (212) 620–0900

Crabtree & Evelyn Ltd. (toiletries, cookies, jams, etc.)
P.O. Box 167
Woodstock Hill, Connecticut 06281 (203) 928–2766

G's Herbs International Ltd. (herbs, teas, spices)
2344 N.W. 21st Place
Portland, Oregon 97210 (503) 241–1131

Hilltop Herb Farm (plants & seeds)
P.O. Box 1734
Cleveland, Texas 77327 (713) 592–5895

Nichols Garden Nursery (plants & seeds)
1190 North Pacific Highway
Albany, Oregon 97321 (503) 928–9280

One Life Natural Foods (dried ingredients & essential oils)
3001 Main Street
Santa Monica, California 90405 (213) 392–4501

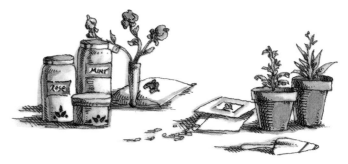

San Francisco Herb Company (dried ingredients)
250 14th Street
San Francisco, California 94103 (415) 861–7174

Star & Crescent Herbs, Inc. (medicinal herbs & colognes)
8561 Thys Court
Sacramento, California 95828 (916) 381–2075

Sunnybrook Farms Nursery (plants & seeds)
9448 Mayfield Road
Chesterland, Ohio 44026 (216) 729–7232

About the Author/Illustrator

Catherine Kanner is an illustrator whose work has appeared in many publications including *The New York Times,* the *Atlantic Monthly, Sports Illustrated, Time, Town and Country,* and *TV Guide.* Each week for the past five years she has drawn an illustration for the Opinion Section of the *Los Angeles Times.* Catherine Kanner lives in Santa Monica, California.

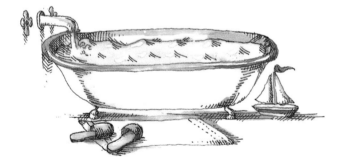

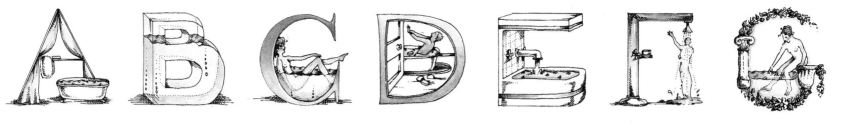

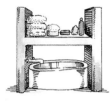 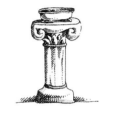 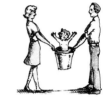 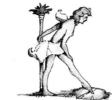 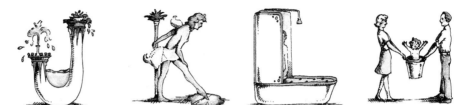 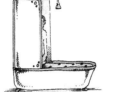 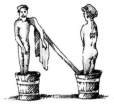

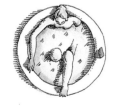 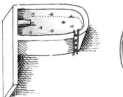 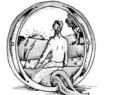 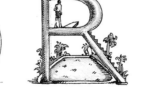 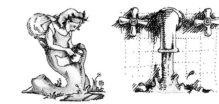 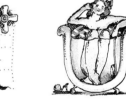

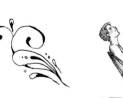 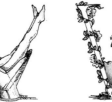 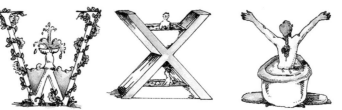 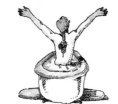 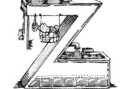